A Post-Graduate's Guide to Doing a Literature Review

A Post-Graduate's Guide to Doing a Literature Review

Third Edition

Helen Aveyard, Sheila Payne and Nancy Preston

Open University Press

Open University Press
McGraw Hill
Unit 4
Foundation Park
Roxborough Way
Maidenhead
SL6 3UD

email: emea_uk_ireland@mheducation.com
world wide web: www.mheducation.co.uk

First published 2016
Second edition published 2021
First published in this third edition 2026

Executive Editor: Sam Crowe
Editorial Assistant: Molly Overend
Content Product Manager: Graham Jones

A catalogue record of this book is available from the British Library

ISBN-13: 9780335253470
ISBN-10: 0335253474
eISBN-13: 9780335253487

Typeset by Transforma Pvt. Ltd., Chennai, India

010288 ACL 2026

Praise for this book

"A Post-Graduate's Guide to Doing a Literature Review in Health and Social Care is an exceptionally clear, practical and confidence-building text for post-graduate students navigating the complexity of literature reviewing. It provides step-by-step guidance on developing focused questions, searching systematically, selecting and appraising evidence, and synthesising findings into a coherent and academically robust review. The third edition is particularly timely in its thoughtful discussion of rigour and the evolving role of AI in the review process. An essential resource for students across health and social care disciplines."

Victoria Sweetmore, Subject Lead, Mental Health and Learning Disability Nursing, University of Derby, UK.

"This third edition covers a range of contemporary issues relevant to literature reviewing in health and social care. Aveyard and colleagues tackle many critical aspects, including the complex and perhaps thorny issue of artificial intelligence. This brings the book right up-to-date and provides an invaluable, core text for post-graduate students."

Dr Caroline Bradbury-Jones, Professor of Gender Based Violence and Health, Department of Nursing and Midwifery, University of Birmingham, UK.

"A Post-Graduate's Guide to Doing a Literature Review in Health and Social Care is an outstanding and trusted resource for post-graduate students and early career researchers. Clear, practical, and methodologically rigorous, this third edition builds on the book's established strengths while remaining highly accessible. Aveyard, Payne and Preston demystify the literature review process, offering step-by-step guidance that is grounded in real research practice. This is an essential companion for anyone undertaking postgraduate study in health and social care and a text I recommend with confidence."

Professor Debra Jackson AO

"The book represents an invaluable resource for students engaged in conducting a literature review. It has also been highly beneficial within my own academic development, offering both clarity and substantive guidance. The writing is consistently well structured, enabling complex information to be accessed and understood with ease. The most recent edition provides an updated and coherent narrative, incorporating current developments and revised referencing that reflect the evolving landscape of the field.

The chapters are organised logically, allowing the text to be read from cover to cover or used to dip into as required. Although the content builds from basic principles, it does not presume prior knowledge, making it suitable for readers at varying stages of study. While certain concepts are complex, they are presented in a manner that remains accessible and engaging. Overall, this book constitutes an essential resource for anyone undertaking a literature review within health and social care."

Christine Rospopa , Assistant Professor, School of Nursing, Midwifery and Health, Coventry University, UK.

"With a scarcity of textbooks on literature reviews at post-graduate level, this unique and fully updated book by Aveyard et al provides a well-informed companion for anyone conducting a systematic review of literature at a professional level. As a step-by-step guide it takes a methodical, yet analytical approach that addresses all components from initial thoughts on conducting a review to the final write-up. Useful to see perspectives on the significance of artificial intelligence, and examples of reviews from a variety of disciplines strengthen this edition of the book as a comprehensive and complete guide."

Dr Neil Gopee, Lecturer in Health and Care, Coventry University, UK.

"Aveyard et al.'s A Post-graduates Guide to doing a Literature Review in Health and Social Care is a highly accessible and practical guide that is particularly well suited to postgraduate students undertaking literature reviews for the first time. One of the book's greatest strengths lies in its clear, straightforward language, which demystifies what is often perceived as a complex and intimidating research task.

The step-by-step approach enhances the book's usability. Each stage of the literature review process is explained in a logical and structured manner. Concepts are introduced gradually, avoiding unnecessary jargon, and technical terms are clearly defined. This makes the text especially beneficial for students from diverse academic or professional backgrounds who may have limited prior research experience.

The practical focus of the book supports student learning. Examples, summary boxes, reflective questions, and case studies are used effectively to reinforce key points and encourage active engagement with the material. These features allow students to directly apply guidance to their own work, enhancing confidence and independence. The writing style remains supportive and instructional throughout, striking a balance between academic rigour and approachability."

Ruth Trout, Senior Lecturer in Acute Care and Continuing Professional Development, Dissertation Supervisor, Buckinghamshire New University, UK.

"A 'Postgraduate's Guide to Doing a Literature Review' is a valuable resource for postgraduate students in nursing and healthcare to develop strong literature-review skills. The textbook offers an accessible overview of core principles, explaining how to approach the process in a robust and systematic way. It encourages students to view the literature review as an engaging and intellectually rewarding part of the research journey. This text is highly recommended for all postgraduate students."

Professor Graeme D. Smith, S. K. Yee School of Health Sciences, Saint Francis University, Hong Kong, SAR, China.

"They say that all good things come in small packages, and this highly respected text is no exception. Whilst the new edition has been refreshed with the welcome inclusion of debate around the use and limitations of Artificial Intelligence, it retains its essential core quality which is its useability. Following the traditional 'what', 'why' and 'how' approach it supports the reader to develop essential knowledge and skills to undertake a literature review without unnecessarily muddying or complicating the process. The content is comprehensive yet presented in a very

straight forward way that will engage even the most reading adverse of students. This text should be essential reading for all students undertaking postgraduate studies in health or social care or undergraduates who wish to further develop their skills in this area."

Dr Helen Atherton, Lecturer in Nursing, University of Leeds, UK.

"Aveyard, Payne & Preston's book is a characteristically highly accessible read for students, comprehensively covering the key aspects of conducting a literature review at postgrad level. It explores different review methods and takes students through the various processes of how to conduct searches, select relevant papers, critically appraise papers, extract data, analyse and synthesise findings, and finally write up and present their review. As such, it is a text I confidently recommend to my postgrad students to use as a guide. I am delighted to see in this latest edition the authors' reflections on AI, insights from international scholars on their choice of review methods, provision of wide-ranging cross-discipline examples, and flagging of additional resources."

Prof Morag Farquhar, University of East Anglia, UK.

Contents

Introduction

We have written this book in order to highlight the importance and relevance of the literature review to your post-graduate project; whether your project is a small-scale study or a larger project at PhD or doctoral level – or somewhere in between. At all levels of post-graduate study, you need to engage with an extensive amount of existing literature, in order to justify, inform and develop your project.

As you start to think about your post-graduate studies, you have already begun to read around your topic and you may have encountered a vast selection of literature – for example, research, discussion, theories, views and opinions. You may be wondering how to make sense of what you are reading and how you might integrate these different types of evidence into your literature review at the level expected of a post-graduate student.

While this can seem daunting, the aim of this book is to guide you through the types of literature you will encounter and the ways these can be integrated into your post-graduate project. We will also describe the different methods of literature review that can be used and help you to identify the one that is most appropriate for your study. You will see that we refer to a variety of methods for conducting a literature review. It is beyond the scope of this book to discuss all the approaches in detail. If you decide to focus in depth on a particular method, we will refer you to further appropriate texts.

Literature reviews are becoming increasingly important in health and social care. This is because there is an increasing amount of published material, which means that it is impossible for a practitioner to keep up to date with every piece of research in his or her area. A literature review therefore provides a summary of the research and other relevant information on a particular research question to inform practice. A literature review is also an essential prerequisite to any empirical study.

Therefore, different projects need different approaches to literature reviewing. Some projects will use the existing literature to justify a larger empirical research study while others will use the existing literature to answer a question without proceeding on to an empirical study. The methods of doing these literature reviews are the same, but there may be a subtle difference in the emphasis of the review, depending on its role in your project (Figure 0.1).

The importance of a rigorous approach to reviewing the literature, rather than simply 'cherry picking' literature that is relevant to your review, prior to an empirical study is increasingly recognized. It is also acknowledged that the literature review can be a study in its own right. The importance of the literature review has been influenced by the emergence of the Cochrane and Campbell Collaborations and their systematic approach to literature reviewing. These collaborations were developed as part of the move towards evidence-based practice, which has challenged practitioners to use the best available evidence to inform their practice. The Cochrane and Campbell Collaborations have drawn attention to the importance of the literature review and, as a result, in many areas of health and social care, there are summaries of evidence to guide practice and online access to systematic reviews, which are published through various professional organizations.

The increasing importance of the literature review within health and social care has led to a re-energizing of the role of the literature

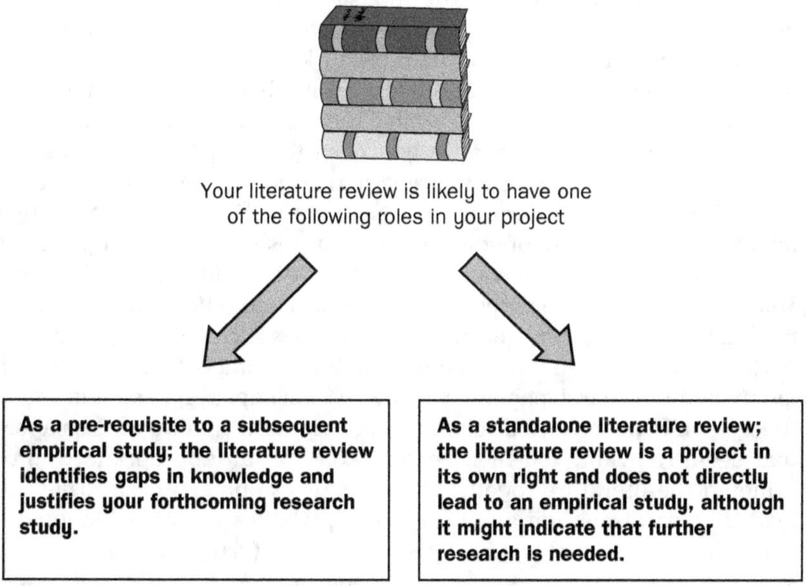

Figure 0.1 Different roles of a literature review

review within post-graduate projects; we argue that the literature review should be regarded as a central component of your project and a research project in its own right, which can be written up and submitted for publication. It is worth noting that a literature review that has been undertaken rigorously is more likely to be accepted for publication as a piece of research in its own right.

In this book, we will discuss the underlying principles for doing a literature review in a robust and systematic manner, and these are principles common to all reviews. This includes how to search and make sense of the literature you find. This will be explained in more depth than you may have considered at under-graduate level. You might be thinking that artificial intelligence (AI) can do this work for you. In our view, this is not possible. Whilst AI can give you a broad summary of some of the existing work that has been undertaken, this is by no means comprehensive or provided with any detail as to the context and quality of the work. The intellectual work required to understand the existing literature is not something that can be replicated by an electronic algorithm. AI can, however, be used to complete some of the tasks required in the review and we will discuss these in the book.

Once you have identified your literature review question(s), your aim usually is to identify all of the published and sometimes unpublished literature that relates to your review question so that you can make a careful judgement about what is already known about your topic. In order to do this, your review should be comprehensive and demonstrate a clear method by which you searched for, and made sense of, the literature you found. This is because you need to be systematic about the approach you take so that you are sure that you have carefully considered all the available literature and have not made vital omissions that might affect the quality of your review. Your research question therefore needs to be clear and to have associated inclusion and exclusion criteria. You need to be able to search for the research and other evidence that is relevant to your review question. You also need to recognize what you find; this might sound like a simple task but it is important that you can distinguish a research paper from a discussion paper or a paper in which theoretical concepts are discussed, and assess the quality of the papers that seem relevant. You then need to consider an appropriate way of bringing the literature together in an analysis and synthesis. This will lead to your discussion and conclusions, which will either highlight a gap in knowledge that can be a justification for further research, or will summarize an existing body of knowledge and hence provide an answer to the question you have set.

You may search for methodological and theoretical literature to support your empirical review. The methodological literature is used to justify your approach to the methods you use in a larger empirical study. The theoretical literature is used to provide an explanatory framework for your empirical review or your eventual empirical findings if you are doing a larger study. Hence you need to identify theories that might be relevant to your research topic.

Rather than approaching the literature review as a necessary and possibly somewhat dull component of your study, we want to encourage you to consider the literature review as a crucial and engaging part of your project that will shape the later stages of your work. Engaging fully with the literature at this stage is necessary in order to get to know the background empirical, methodological and theoretical work that has been done in your area. It is not possible to start a project at post-graduate level without being aware of others' work because you need to demonstrate the originality of your research question and explain what your study contributes to the overall body of knowledge on a topic. You need this background analysis of the literature in order to 'pick up the baton' from other researchers, whose work will inform your project in many ways.

In this book, we will discuss the different features of the literature review:

- In Chapter 1 we will discuss what a literature review is and why it is important in your post-graduate project.
- In Chapter 2 we will discuss the different types of literature reviews.
- In Chapter 3 we will discuss the inclusion of theoretical, methodological and empirical literature in a literature review and will discuss the role of the research question in shaping the review.
- In Chapter 4 we will discuss how to develop a thorough search strategy that goes beyond simple database searching.
- In Chapter 5 we will discuss how to identify what is relevant to your literature review from the data you have gathered.
- In Chapter 6 we will discuss the role of critical appraisal of the research and other evidence, and how critical appraisal can be incorporated into the literature review, according to the approach you are following.
- In Chapter 7 we will discuss how to analyse and synthesize the research and other evidence you have, according to the requirements of the approach to literature review you are following.
- In Chapter 8 we will discuss how to write up your findings and present your literature review.

What's new in this third edition

As researchers and academics, we follow the developments and trends in methods for doing a literature review closely. We have refreshed the text by incorporating the latest nuanced developments and ideas into this new edition. For this edition, we have included our reflections on the ways that AI is influencing the way we do literature reviews and our thoughts about using AI whilst still maintaining rigour in a review. In addition, we have developed discussion around the various types of literature reviews and have obtained the rationale from scholars around the world as to why they undertook their study in the way that they did. We have also included a wide range of examples from different disciplines to reinforce the arguments throughout the book and have signposted the reader to additional resources where the remit of the discussion lays outside this textbook.

1

What is a literature review?

In this chapter, we will discuss:

- *What a literature review is*
- *The common features of a literature review*
- *Why a literature review is important in your post-graduate project*
- *The role a literature review plays in your project*
- *The importance of a focused question for your review.*

What is a literature review?

A literature review is an analysis and synthesis of work that has been undertaken in a particular area: the area that most closely relates to the research question you are exploring for your post-graduate study, be it a small-scale study, master's or a PhD or doctoral-level award. A literature review involves identifying a question (or questions), which is then answered by the comprehensive and systematic identification, analysis and synthesis of a relevant body of published and sometimes unpublished research and other evidence. The aim of a literature review is to identify what we know and do not know about the question identified. There are many different types of literature review and we will refer to the complexity surrounding this throughout the book. Some are reductive and seek to summarize the available information while others are interpretive and seek to generate understanding. The principles we review in this book apply to all literature reviews; the level of detail to which you apply them will depend on the scope of your individual study.

Literature reviews have become increasingly popular in recent years due to the vast amount of published research and other information associated with the emphasis on evidence-based practice. A literature review aims to make sense of a body of research and other evidence, and presents a summary and analysis of this so that the reader does not have to access and read each individual research report or other material included in the review. This is important because there are increasing amounts of publications and other sources of information available, and it is an impossible task to read and assimilate all the information on any one topic. In addition, a well-conducted literature review will provide a critique of the identified research and other evidence and may not include that which is considered to be of poorer quality. This means that when the literature is synthesized together, it is possible to draw conclusions about all the relevant and better-quality research and other evidence. This reduces the likelihood that one misleading research paper will dominate readers' attention and should prevent a 'rogue' piece of evidence from taking centre stage (Harden and Thomas 2005).

Some researchers have commented on the risk that individual pieces of literature, in particular qualitative research studies, are stripped of their context when they are summarized and included in a literature review. These concerns are noted by Thomas and Harden (2008), Noblit and Hare (1988), Pawson et al. (2005) and Sandelowski et al. (1997) and this can be exacerbated by reviews that are not well conducted (Page and Moher 2016; Thorne 2017). However, there is also recognition that without bringing research and other evidence together in a review, individual pieces of research cannot be seen in the context of others. Most researchers agree that bringing the research and other evidence together in a review is a necessary and highly useful task, and the utility of bringing a body of literature together outweighs some of the inevitable 'context stripping'.

There are many different approaches to literature reviewing, which we will discuss throughout this book. Reviews can be composed of all types of published and unpublished research and other material – whatever is relevant to answering the review question.

The common features of a literature review

Although there are many approaches to conducting a literature review, they share many common attributes. If you are undertaking a literature review for a post-graduate award, then the aim of your review will be to present a summary and synthesis of the relevant literature relating to the focus of your specific literature review question(s). While there are many nuances, the overall principles that you will adhere to are generally those listed below:

Features that are common to most literature reviews

- Focused literature review question
- Inclusion and exclusion criteria
- Specific key words and terms
- List of databases and other sources of evidence
- Record of searches undertaken
- Data extraction in a similar manner from all included papers
- Critique and assessment of design and conduct of all research literature included
- Presentation of data from all papers
- Analysis and synthesis of the findings in relation to the research question
- Discussion of the extent to which the research question has been answered
- Identification of what is known and what remains unknown
- Standardized method of reporting the review.

A clear focus is vital and this is usually achieved by defining a review question (or questions) and related inclusion and exclusion criteria, which determine the remit of the review. Without this, there is a good chance that the focus of the review will 'drift' as interesting but unrelated literature is uncovered. Inclusion and exclusion criteria will enable you to identify research or other evidence that is directly related to answering your review question. Literature that does not meet these criteria can be discarded or be retained in case it provides useful background information.

Searching for relevant research and other evidence is a key aspect in all literature reviews. Reviewers will generally identify key terms that capture the essence of the question they have identified together with a list of potential electronic databases on which to search; however, searching is not limited to a database search. The main focus of the search is likely to be empirical research but you will need to search for other evidence, including methodological and theoretical literature, especially if your literature review is for a doctoral or PhD study. In most cases, the reviewer is searching for all the relevant research that meets the inclusion criteria so that the review is comprehensive and does not make vital omissions. We will discuss this further in Chapter 4.

The search for research and other evidence will inevitably lead you to a wide range of literature and you will need to extract what is relevant for your review, according to the inclusion and exclusion criteria you have identified. Not all of the aspects of all the research or other evidence will be relevant to you and you need to identify what is. There are data extraction (summary) forms that you can develop to assist this process, which we will discuss in Chapter 5.

Once the relevance of the research or other evidence has been established, there are considerations of quality to be made. The literature is likely to be of varying quality and you will need to make a judgement about it and the impact that it will have in your subsequent analysis. This is an area where many methodological differences arise, both in the methods of assessing quality and the decision about the inclusion of research of different qualities in your review. There can be a lack of agreement about what amounts to quality in both the design and conduct of research. For these reasons, it is not always easy to establish the quality of the research or other evidence you have. However, this assessment needs to be made and a judgement is needed, as you will generally give more weight to the better designed and conducted research in your subsequent analysis and synthesis. There are also different views on the inclusion of literature of different quality. Some literature reviews include all research that is considered relevant while other reviews exclude research on the basis of their quality. Therefore, you may sometimes use lower-quality research if you make the judgement about how and when to include it. If you do not include lower-quality research, you need to justify your decision to exclude it. We will discuss this in Chapter 6. You can determine the strength of evidence most easily if you use an appropriate critical appraisal tool. Appraisal tools are available for virtually all types of evidence that are relevant to your review. We will also discuss this in Chapter 6.

Once you have identified the quality and relevance of the research and other evidence, you need to combine them in an analysis and synthesis of the studies using a suitable method for your review. Data analysis and synthesis are common to all literature reviews, but this is another area where many methodological differences arise. The approach taken will depend on the type of review. If the included research papers are sufficiently similar and use statistics, this can be done numerically, using a statistical calculation often referred to as a meta-analysis. When a meta-analysis is not possible or appropriate, the research or other evidence can be analysed using a non-numerical narrative approach. This generally involves a form of thematic analysis and there are many approaches to this, including meta-synthesis, meta-ethnography and thematic analysis. Those of you doing a scoping review will focus on providing an overview of the available evidence rather than a critical analysis. Munn et al. (2018) provide a useful discussion about this and we will address the matter further in Chapter 7.

Finally, there should be a structured and transparent reporting of the process of undertaking the review and of the results so that what is known and what remains unknown is clearly communicated and set in the context of your ongoing study. We will discuss this in Chapter 8.

Why is a literature review important for my post-graduate project?

The literature review is important for your post-graduate project because, at this level of study, it is essential that you consider what other academic work exists in the area you are researching and what the strengths and limitations of this work are. It is important that you acknowledge that your work does not exist in isolation, and that you can demonstrate how your work relates to the work of others and the contribution of your project to the overall body of knowledge, however modest you consider that to be. You need to come to a conclusion about the contribution made by the existing body of literature to your understanding of your research question. In short, you cannot build your own project without building on the work of others.

However large or small your post-graduate study, you need to consider all the evidence that is relevant to your area of work in a comprehensive and systematic manner. This will be the case whether your entire post-graduate study is literature based or whether you will be reviewing the literature before or after undertaking your own empirical study.

Undertaking a structured review is important in order to ensure that you do not overlook a piece of literature that is relevant to your research question in your review. Students are often concerned that they will attend the oral examination or presentation of their work to find that they have omitted a seminal or very significant piece of work from their literature review. This scenario will be far less likely if you have undertaken a review following a structured approach as we have outlined in the previous section.

Why is there an increasing emphasis on the literature review within my project?

In the last few years, the literature review has been recognized as increasingly important within health and social care generally. We have systematic reviews and summaries of reviews available in clinical practice and online. This is largely in response to the emphasis on evidence-based practice, the increased amount of research publications and the recognition that, in order to be useful, evidence needs to be assimilated and summarized.

As recognition of the importance of the literature review has increased, so has its role within post-graduate study. In the past, a literature review might have been viewed as something to 'get done' in order to get onto the more interesting task of your own research study. There has been an increased focus on the importance of literature reviews either as a prerequisite to and therefore shaping an empirical study, or as the main component of the research study itself. Alongside this is the development of a variety of methods that have been designed for conducting the review. We would encourage all those undertaking a literature review at post-graduate level to consider their method very carefully and to be able to justify the approach they have taken. The process of undertaking a literature review is recognized as a piece of research, and the methods of doing so have become as robust as an empirical research study (Whittemore and Knafl 2005; O'Mathuna 2010; Aveyard 2023).

This has not always been the case. If you have accessed master's dissertations and doctoral theses undertaken in previous decades, you are likely to have found a less standardized approach to literature searching and evaluation. You would have generally found a chapter on 'the literature review' but with probably little or no discussion about how the literature search, appraisal and synthesis were undertaken, or why certain papers were selected for review (Dixon-Woods et al. 2007). Research and development in this area have led to an increased understanding of – and different approaches to – undertaking a literature review, together with an acknowledgement that different types of literature reviews are appropriate for different research questions and that rigour can be achieved whichever review method is undertaken.

The influence of the Cochrane Collaboration on the development of the literature review method

One of the most influential factors on the development of research methods for the literature review has been the work of the Cochrane Collaboration. Whether or not the type of literature review you undertake for your project is similar to a 'Cochrane-style' review, this highly systematic approach to the literature review is likely to have influenced the development of the method of review that you undertake.

The Cochrane Collaboration was founded in 1992 in Oxford, largely due to the influence of epidemiologist Professor Archie Cochrane (1909–1988). Cochrane was one of the first medical scientists to demonstrate the lack of good evidence upon which many medical treatments and interventions were based. He argued that too much remained unknown about the effectiveness of many treatments and interventions (Cochrane 1972) and proclaimed: 'it is surely a great criticism of our profession [medicine] that we have not organised a critical summary of all relevant randomised controlled trials' (Cochrane 1979: 2).

Cochrane challenged the medical community to develop summaries of evidence that would provide guidance for the treatments and interventions given. This challenge resulted in the foundation of the Cochrane Collaboration, which seeks to publish reviews of evidence on the effectiveness of many well-established treatments and interventions. It also provides guidance on the cost-effectiveness of treatments and interventions. This work has brought huge developments in the way we manage health care and is ongoing and thriving today. It has also led to the development of the sister organization, the Campbell Collaboration, founded in 2000, which focuses on systematic reviews with a social policy emphasis. The Campbell Collaboration is named after David Campbell, who was a member of the National Academy of Science in the United States and who advocated that social policy should be based on sound scientific experimentation.

Examples

One early systematic review demonstrated how the standardized review process can provide potentially life-saving information. Mulrow (1994) described a systematic review of 33 studies that looked at the effectiveness of streptokinase in the treatment of acute myocardial infarction (heart attack). Streptokinase, although now well known as a life-saving drug, was at that time not routinely administered to patients following a myocardial infarction due to lack of evidence about its effectiveness. There were many small randomized controlled trials (RCTs) that compared the outcomes of patients who were given streptokinase and those who were not, but the results were inconclusive due to the size of the studies. However, when the results of these studies were pooled in a meta-analysis (a statistical procedure that combines the results of all similar studies), the true effect of the streptokinase became apparent, which had not been identifiable prior to the meta-analysis. This review revolutionized care of patients following myocardial infarction, and Mulrow commented that this benefit could have been demonstrated 20 years previously (and saved many lives) if the meta-analysis had been undertaken much earlier.

Another early systematic review that revolutionized practice was that of Gilbert et al. (2005), who undertook a systematic review that identified equally life-saving information. This team of researchers reviewed the evidence about widely held beliefs that babies should sleep on their stomachs. This public health advice, which had been published in many popular child health textbooks, dated back to the 1960s. In reviewing available research, the researchers found evidence that this advice was incorrect. Gilbert et al. estimate that as many as 10,000 babies' lives could have been saved if an earlier systematic review of this evidence had been undertaken.

As you can see from the examples above, Cochrane systematic reviews with meta-analysis are concerned with determining the effectiveness of treatments and care procedures. They are often composed of randomized controlled trials (RCTs) and reflect a positivist deductive paradigm where results of studies can be compared using statistical techniques. It is widely agreed that if you are concerned with the effectiveness of an intervention, then the best way to find out about it is to undertake an RCT. For this reason, most Cochrane Collaboration systematic reviews incorporate RCTs. Other literature reviews that have a different focus will incorporate a variety of research designs.

What is a randomized controlled trial?

This is an approach to an experiment in which one intervention is compared against another or no intervention. Participants who have agreed to enter an experiment are allocated at random into one of two or more groups. The different groups receive a different treatment or intervention. At the end of the experiment, the effect of each intervention or treatment on the participants in each group is assessed and the differences in outcomes between the participants in different groups compared. The principle is that, due to the random assignment of the treatment, all other influencing factors will be equalled out and any difference between the participants in the different groups can be put down to the different treatments or interventions.

Randomized controlled trials have less systematic bias about the effects of an intervention or treatment and the data can be analysed statistically. For this reason, RCTs are generally used to answer research questions about the effect of an intervention or treatment (for example, the effect of a drug or sleeping position). Although there is general agreement that this type of experiment is the best way to determine whether or not a treatment or intervention is effective, in any health or social care discipline, some researchers argue that there should be an element of caution about this approach. For example, many researchers (e.g. Borgerson 2009; Greenhalgh 2014; Barratt et al. 2016; Minary et al. 2019) have expressed caution about the use of simple experiments to evaluate complex interventions and, when they are, this can lead to the over-simplification of results. This concern reinforced the need for a wide range of research methods to match the question needing to be answered and a corresponding wider range of literature review methods.

Systematic approach to a wider range of literature review questions

Cochrane systematic reviews with a meta-analysis follow a very detailed method, which we will refer to throughout the book. The method is appropriate for summarizing and combining the results of RCTs, when considering the effectiveness of treatments. The interest in and development of the Cochrane Collaboration systematic review has led to greater interest in a more systematic approach to literature reviews more generally, that is, reviews that have a broader remit than determining the effectiveness of treatments. This has led to an expansion of ideas and approaches to comprehensive and systematic reviews of the literature, a lot of which might come from different research paradigms. Hence these methods may differ from the original Cochrane Collaboration approach but the overall aims and intentions will be similar (Grant and Booth 2009; Tong et al. 2012; Aveyard and Bradbury-Jones 2019).

The discussion and focus on the importance of the literature review have re-energized the process of undertaking a literature review, particularly at post-graduate level, and we will discuss a number of different methods throughout this book. What is important is that the researcher develops a systematic and comprehensive approach to the search, appraisal, analysis and synthesis of the research and other material, within the scope that his or her study allows. This should include reference to rigour, transparency and replicability of the method of undertaking the literature review.

Clarification of terminology

There are many different approaches to doing a literature review. Aveyard and Bradbury-Jones (2019) and Sutton et al. (2019) comment on a proliferation of named approaches for doing a review. You can see from the stages discussed on page 3 that most literature reviews follow a systematic and comprehensive approach. Possibly the most comprehensive approach is the systematic review, which is a specific method of undertaking a literature review which we discuss later in this chapter. Clarity about the use of terms is important. All literature reviews should follow a systematic approach and you are encouraged to adopt a systematic approach to any type of literature review you embark on. In other words, your review will be systematic even if it does not adhere to the detail of what is formally referred to as a systematic review and may, in fact, be more closely aligned with another method of review. The point to remember is that your review should be done systematically, whether or not you are specifically undertaking a systematic review.

You might also find that the term 'meta-analysis' – a term used to refer to the statistical analysis of the results from individual research studies within a systematic review – is used to describe a systematic review that includes a meta-analysis (Saba et al. 2014).

What role will a literature review play in my project?

There are many different roles that the literature review might play and many different types of literature review methods that you could use. This will depend on your individual research project and you will establish the role of your literature review in your study during discussion with your supervisor or supervisory team. For most research projects at post-graduate level, the literature review will fall into one of two categories (Table 1.1):

- Supportive literature review
- Standalone literature review.

Do remember that whichever type of review you undertake for your post-graduate studies, you can consider publication of your review. This is especially relevant to (though not restricted) PhD-level study where a publication provides evidence that your work has been subject to peer review.

Table 1.1 The role of the literature review in your research project

	The research question is answered **by a comprehensive and systematic literature review**	**The research project is** supported **by a comprehensive and systematic literature review**
Your main project is an empirical study. The literature review will consider what we already know about the topic and justify your research question. We will refer to this as a **supportive literature review**		✓
Your main project is a literature review from which you hope to answer a research question. We will refer to this as a **standalone literature review**	✓	

Supportive literature review

This is the classic approach to the literature review. It is undertaken prior to an empirical study, often as part of a PhD or master's or a much larger funded study. The purpose of the literature review is to inform the researchers of all relevant previous work that has been done in that area. This will often focus on what other empirical research has been undertaken in the area but will also draw on other types of literature, such as theoretical and methodological literature. It helps to identify what is known and what is unknown about the topic of your research. There is a caveat here, however, as in certain approaches to qualitative research – for example, grounded theory – the literature review may be undertaken after the main study has been completed so as not to influence or lead the initial analysis.

Standalone literature review

This is a more recent type of literature review in which the intention of the review is to answer a research question rather than to identify a gap in knowledge that leads to further research, although these reviews often do point to the need for further research. The methods for undertaking this approach have been the focus of much scrutiny in recent years due to the attention given to this method by the Cochrane Collaboration and the development of the systematic review. While not all literature reviews that attempt to address a research question as their main purpose use a Cochrane-style systematic review method, most strive for a systematic approach. This type of review is helpful when you need to evaluate the contribution of the existing literature to knowledge in a particular area, such as the most appropriate interventions or services to commission.

The importance of a focused literature review question

Whatever role the literature review plays in your research, it is important that your research is led by a focused question. If there are several sections to your literature review, each is likely to be led by a different question, which will have a specific focus. Therefore, it is important to identify a focused literature review question so that the aims and scope of your review are clear from the outset. This might sound obvious, but one of the common pitfalls for those undertaking a literature review is a lack of clarity about the aims and purpose of the review. This is important as otherwise you will risk going 'off track' and including literature that is interesting but irrelevant to the aims of your review. Many students commence their literature review lacking clarity about what they need to achieve and hence fail to include the most appropriate research or other evidence and subsequently waste a lot of time and effort. Without a clear question, there is also the risk that you will drift from the main aims of the review while the review is in progress. As a result, the review might be vague and not meet the needs of the project.

Associated with the development of a clear question is the development of clear inclusion and exclusion criteria that provide a detailed guide to the literature that will be relevant to your review. Inclusion and exclusion criteria allow you as the researcher to be very specific about the type of literature you will include. We will discuss this further when we discuss searching for literature in Chapter 4.

Sometimes the literature review question will be a simple deductive question. This assumes that the 'answer' can be found in research or other evidence by a simple deductive process. The terms used to describe the literature review question are likely to be unambiguous and clearly defined in the existing work available. For example, a literature review question might seek to find out about evidence of the effectiveness of topical antibiotics in treating impetigo in young children.

For most literature review questions, it is important that you can define the terms used in the literature review question. In this case, the terms 'effectiveness' and 'young children' would need to be clearly defined so that the researcher is clear about the focus of the review and that this clarity is then present in the review.

At times, however, the purpose of the literature review will be to clarify and develop concepts (Dixon-Woods et al. 2005). For these types of review, it may not be possible to clearly define the terms used at the outset, which might initially be 'tentative, fuzzier and contested' (Greenhalgh et al. 2005: 418). A concept analysis is an example of an approach to reviewing published material in order to clarify the working use of a term (Rodgers 1989, 2000). For example, a literature review question might seek to consider how a concept is discussed in published material. Autonomy is an example of a concept that might mean different things to different people and so is not easy to define, and it was the subject of a concept analysis undertaken by Lindberg et al. (2014).

The role that your literature review plays in your project might have an influence on the literature review question. If your main project is a standalone literature review and you intend to answer a specific question through an analysis of the research and other relevant evidence, then the focus of your literature review question is likely to be the same as the focus of your entire project. While you are also likely to refer to the methodological literature to justify the approach you took in the design of your review and the theoretical literature in order to develop the theories that relate to your review, the main focus of your review will be the literature that directly answers your literature review question.

If your main project is an empirical study, your study is likely to be supported by one or more literature reviews – for example, an empirical literature review of what is already known about the focus of your study, in addition to a review of theoretical and empirical literature relating to different aspects of the research question and how it is going to be answered. Each of these sections is likely to have a different question.

The important point is that your literature review must be focused around a specific question that is relevant for your project. Your question will be supported by inclusion and exclusion criteria that will guide your search for relevant research and other information, which we will discuss in Chapter 4.

In summary

In this chapter, we have described what a literature review is and the common features that are associated with most reviews. We have also described the role that a literature review might play in your post-graduate study. At the start of your review, you need to identify whether your literature review will be a standalone review or a prerequisite to a larger empirical study, and this may have a subtle effect on the way you approach your review, as portrayed in Table 1.1. It is vital to have a clearly focused question for your literature review, otherwise the review is likely to become unfocused. The research question and associated inclusion and exclusion criteria will direct the focus of the review.

We have argued that the importance of the literature review in your post-graduate project has increased in recent years and that this is related to the increased importance and significance of the role of the literature review within health and social care more generally. While it has always been important to set your work within the context of others', the methods of doing so have recently become more diverse, explicit and rigorous. In the next chapter, we will discuss the different approaches to undertaking a literature review.

Key points

- A literature review is an analysis and synthesis of work undertaken in an area
- It is important to set your work within the context of others'
- The methods for undertaking a literature review have developed in recent years
- There are features that are common to most literature reviews
- Your review might be a standalone review or supportive to a larger study
- It is important to have a clearly focused question for your review.

2

Different methods for doing a literature review

In this chapter, we will discuss:

- *Different methods of doing a literature review*
- *Examples of projects where different methods have been used.*

Once you have established the role that the literature review will play in your study and the focus of your literature review question, you need to consider the most appropriate method for your review. There are many different types of literature review methods. Some are concerned with the synthesis of quantitative research, others with examining qualitative research, and still others a combination of the two. Some use qualitative methods of analysis and synthesis and others use quantitative statistical methods.

There is no one type of literature review method that is better than another (Arksey and O'Malley 2005) and most can be conducted with a rigorous method; you should choose the one that best fits the literature and the study and you must be ready to defend your choice in your written dissertation or viva. Some reviews reflect a Cochrane-style systematic review with meta-analysis while others take a more narrative approach. The approach that you take will depend on your project and we will discuss this later in this chapter. There are also some that can be undertaken by novice researchers and others that are recommended for those with more expertise. For example, some of the approaches to reviewing the literature require a team of researchers to complete, such as using a detailed systematic review method like that undertaken by the Cochrane Collaboration. However, there are ways that you can adapt these approaches and we will explore how potentially complex methods can be adapted and used appropriately and realistically for post-graduate study. An important point to remember is that, at whatever level you are writing your literature review, you can undertake a comprehensive and systematic approach that is relevant for the project you are doing.

Different approaches to your literature review

In this section, we will discuss a range of approaches you might consider using, depending on the needs of your study and the role that the literature review plays in your research. Any of these approaches can be used whether your literature review is a standalone study or a prerequisite to a larger study, although the time and word limit you have for your review will influence the approach you take and the detail with which you are able to carry out the review. You may follow one of the methods we describe in this chapter, or you may follow the general principles of a literature review without adhering to a specific method. If you decide to focus on one of the approaches in a larger-scale review, we advise that you access the additional references we have given, which fully describe the method. Some of the approaches can be used for the review of empirical research only, while others combine the review of empirical, theoretical and other literature.

We have created Table 2.1 to try and categorize different types of reviews. Some reviews can be assigned into more than one category – for example, we have allocated narrative synthesis into theory driven but it could be used in qualitative evidence synthesis or even as a method to describe results of a quantitative review which was not suitable for a meta-analysis. This list is by no means exhaustive but represents a range of review types. Do note that all review types might be prefixed using the term ‘systematic’.

Table 2.1 A selection of different types of literature reviews

1

Systematic reviews with meta-analysis:
This is the original systematic review of quantitative research. The aim is a meta-analysis or statistical re-analysis of the results of included papers which can be supplemented by a quantitative synthesis. When a meta-analysis is not appropriate, a narrative synthesis (usually qualitative) might be undertaken

2

Descriptive mapping reviews:
Incorporating quantitative and qualitative research where findings are pooled together but little further analysis is undertaken: meta-aggregation or scoping review

3

Qualitative evidence synthesis:
Incorporating qualitative research where findings are combined and re-interpreted: meta-ethnography, thematic synthesis

4

Integrative reviews:
Incorporating different types of research where results are re-interpreted: integrative review, mixed-methods review

5

Paradigm or theory-driven reviews:
Incorporating different types of research where the aim is the development of theory: narrative synthesis, realist review, critical interpretive synthesis

(continued)

Table 2.1 Continued

6

Overview of reviews:
Incorporating multiple pre-existing reviews in one overall review: umbrella review, review of reviews

1 Systematic reviews with meta-analysis

We will start with the original systematic review method. We call this the 'original systematic review' because the first systematic reviews were designed to include a meta-analysis, or statistical analysis, of the results of all the included studies in order to determine the effectiveness of a treatment or intervention as discussed earlier. Since then, systematic reviews have developed to include a variety of methods of analysis, but systematic review with a meta-analysis was the original design of this type of review.

The method for undertaking a systematic review with meta-analysis is described and available online in the Cochrane Collaboration Handbook, which was first published in 1994. In this and subsequent editions, the exacting methods of undertaking a Cochrane-style systematic review with meta-analysis have been developed and established, and they are well documented in the latest edition of the handbook (Higgins et al. 2024).

A systematic review with a meta-analysis is a very structured process. It is usually undertaken by a review team so that more than one person performs each task to enhance the accuracy and reliability of the process. The researchers may be assisted by an advisory group, which can include patient and client representatives.

A systematic review aims to identify, evaluate and undertake a statistical re-analysis of data from all the existing studies that refer to a specific research question and that meet specific inclusion and exclusion criteria. For those undertaking a Cochrane systematic review with meta-analysis, the literature review question is usually focused on the effectiveness of an intervention. Other systematic reviews or meta-analyses may have a focus other than that of effectiveness.

One main feature of a systematic review is the effort that is expended in identifying relevant studies for inclusion. The search goes far beyond electronic subject-specific database searches and extends to the location of unpublished papers and other evidence, which we discuss in detail in Chapter 4. The focus of the review is tightly controlled; studies that are interesting but not relevant are often excluded from the review. Studies are assessed for bias; most systematic review protocols have criteria for assessment of bias, which means that those studies that are relevant but of high risk of bias are excluded from the review. It is possible for researchers to identify many studies that are relevant only to reject these studies a little further down the line due to concern about the quality of their design and/or conduct. It is therefore common for researchers to conclude that there is insufficient evidence to answer the research question they set out to address in their systematic review.

The design of the review is written up in advance of performing it, in a protocol that might be published or registered with a register of systematic reviews such as PROSPERO (https://www.crd.york.ac.uk/prospero/). Protocols ensure transparency and if more than one person is involved with the review, it helps to ensure that everyone is following the same steps. There are many excellent texts that report in detail the process of undertaking a systematic review (Centre for Reviews and Dissemination 2008; Bettany-Saltikov 2012; Chandler and Hopewell 2013; Higgins et al. 2024).

Understanding the impact of systematic reviews

The systematic review with meta-analysis is generally viewed to be one of the greatest scientific advances of our time. It has enabled scientists and the medical community to state with more certainty what does and what does not work, or what is effective and what is not, in terms of treatments and screening interventions, thus helping decision-making for screening and treatment options. However, the process is not necessarily straightforward. In 2011, the Nordic Cochrane group published a systematic review in which their analysis showed that mammograms were not effective in reducing the mortality rate from breast cancer (Gotzsche and Nielsen 2011). These findings provoked intense discussion among scientists and the medical community, and when the papers were re-analysed, omitting some of the older papers from the meta-analysis (Marmot et al. 2012), the results were more consistent with previous recommendations. Hence it remains a judgement call as to which studies are included in the analysis and the consequences of this.

Even if we accept the need for informed judgement, more fundamentally, the systematic review and the randomized controlled trial (RCT), which is often selected within a systematic review, are not without their critics. For example, Seers (2007) expresses concern that data might not be as context free as we might like to think and that results from RCTs might imply a robustness of the results that may not exist in reality. Pawson et al. (2005) are particularly critical of systematic reviews that attempt to combine data in a meta-analysis from disparate studies. They argue that unless studies are conducted in exceptionally similar settings, with similar context and participants, the results cannot be meaningfully pooled in a meta-analysis. However, the Cochrane Collaboration do not recommend that results are just a pooled estimate of effect. Instead, they require a narrative critique of the included papers together with an acknowledgement of the limitations of pooling results, such as the level of heterogeneity (or differences) between participants or interventions.

Example of systematic reviews with meta-analysis

We contacted the authors of a systematic review and meta-analysis on 'Interventions to improve nurses' job satisfaction' (Niskala et al. 2020). In an email correspondence, Kristina Mikkonen (2020) told us: '*The systematic review is a rigid systematic method of evidence identification, screening process, and quality evaluation. The PICOS format inclusion and exclusion criteria supported each researcher in their screening process. The screening process was conducted among the three researchers by reading 489 titles, 61 abstracts, and 47 full-text articles. The process was done by each researcher first separately and later agreed together. The meta-analysis was selected to measure the effectiveness of these interventions. Our systematic review found evidence-based knowledge, which will be relevant for decision-making regarding nurse satisfaction in healthcare organizations. For instance, we found in our meta-analysis that among 20 different types of interventions, only two interventions significantly improved nurses' job satisfaction*'.

When might a systematic review with meta-analysis be appropriate for your post-graduate study?

A systematic review with meta-analysis may be appropriate if you are reviewing studies using quantitative designs that fulfil the criteria to be combined in a meta-analysis. Systematic reviews with a meta-analysis have been undertaken at PhD or doctoral-level study and sometimes at master's-level work, and the process can be adapted to suit your level of experience and resources. For example, the role of the team of researchers and advisory group usually associated with a systematic review project can be carried out by members of your supervisory team, and peers or colleagues may be prepared to become involved with your work and assist you in making decisions about the conduct of your systematic review, thus enhancing its rigour. It is therefore advisable to find at least one academic within your discipline who is willing to duplicate some of the tasks you need to carry out when undertaking the review, as this will increase the accuracy of your review and make it more publishable. We will discuss the tasks where this is possible throughout this book.

For example, Labrague and Cayaban (2025) undertook a systematic review and meta-analysis to examine the association between hospital patient safety culture and missing nursing care. Their review highlighted important implications for nurse managers on the importance of fostering an effective patient safety culture including education and policies.

Systematic review with a narrative synthesis

In addition to a meta-analysis, a quantitative narrative synthesis – to be distinguished from the mixed-methods approach to narrative synthesis discussed later in this chapter – can be used. One of the first articulations of this approach (Popay et al. 2006; Pope et al. 2007) is narrative synthesis: the description, explanation and interpretation of the study findings and the attempt to find explanations for the findings, which enhance or replace the interpretation of the meta-analysis. In a quantitative narrative synthesis, the results of the systematic review are described rather than numerically analysed. There is a focus on the context and study characteristics in order to develop a richer, more in-depth understanding of the results than that presented in the statistics provided by the meta-analysis. Recently, this approach has been developed by Campbell et al. (2020), who articulate methods for analysing data where a meta-analysis is not possible. Campell et al. refer to these methods as 'synthesis without meta-analysis', or SWiM, bringing transparency and a clear method for those who analyse data when a meta-analysis is not possible.

Alternative types of systematic reviews

The term systematic review is not reserved exclusively for reviews produced by the Cochrane or Campbell Collaboration, and systematic reviews are often undertaken to address literature review questions that do not address questions of effectiveness. However, there is ongoing debate as to whether alternative approaches to undertaking a review should be referred to as systematic reviews as has been discussed in Chapter 1 (Aveyard and Bradbury-Jones 2019). As a result, there are a range of terms used to describe literature review, some using the prefix 'systematic' and others not.

When a systematic review with a meta-analysis is not appropriate for your study – for example, you may have data which are insufficient for the calculation of effect sizes, or you have qualitative studies or a wide range of qualitative and quantitative research – there are many other approaches to (systematic) literature review that you can consider. Your decision will depend on the types of papers that you have and the level of analysis you intend to undertake.

Most of these approaches contain the common features of a literature review as presented in Chapter 1; however, there are many subtle differences that you will take into account if you follow one of these methods. The different methods of literature review vary according to the methods of searching, critical appraisal and analysis. Some reviews aim to pool and combine the results reported in the literature and summarize what the different studies are saying, while others aim for interpretation.

2 Descriptive mapping reviews

A descriptive, mapping approach to doing a review is a systematic approach to summarizing the available literature. It provides a systematic and comprehensive overview but does not intend to re-interpret or analyse findings.

Scoping review

A scoping review is an approach that incorporates all types of research and other evidence in a review (Arksey and O'Malley 2005). This is a versatile and flexible approach to a review, the aim of which is to map key areas of research or the use of concepts – for example, how particular terms are used and for what purposes (Mays et al. 2005). Scoping studies can be the precursor to a detailed literature review and are generally less detailed than the other literature review methods referred to in this chapter. A scoping study will usually involve the identification of a research question and broad searching strategy, followed by the charting and summarizing of the data. Literature is not generally omitted from the review according to quality criteria and there is no attempt to weight the evidence. According to Arksey and O'Malley, 'this is because the scoping study does not seek to assess the quality of evidence and consequently cannot determine whether particular studies provide robust and generalizable findings' (2005: 27). Literature is summarized rather than synthesized. The authors argue:

> *the scoping study does not address the issue of synthesis, that is the relative weight of evidence in favour of the effectiveness of any particular intervention ... consequently scoping studies provide a narrative or descriptive account of available research.*
>
> (Arksey and O'Malley 2005: 30)

When might a scoping review be appropriate for your post-graduate study?

A scoping study is a useful first step if you are undertaking a large-scale project such as a PhD or doctoral study. It can then be used as a basis for a more in-depth literature review as your project progresses. It provides an overview of the volume of published work on a topic and may help to guide a subsequent more selective review. Webster et al. (2020) undertook a scoping review of the technology to support the emotional and social well-being of nurses. In an email correspondence, Natalie Webster (2020) explained why this was an appropriate method:

> *I really liked the idea of a scoping review as a 'reconnaissance exercise'; which can be used where there is limited published material in the research topic, and also as a means of investigating if a full systematic review would be worthwhile for a future study. At this stage we were not ready to undertake a systematic review, which would have needed a more focused research question; the broad nature of our enquiry really suited a scoping review methodology. I think in the end, a narrative approach to a scoping review really suited our aims and enabled us to compare and contrast a variety of academic and grey literature from a diverse range of disciplines which used technology to support nurses, midwives, students and patients.*

Meta-aggregation

The meta-aggregative review was developed by researchers at the Joanna Briggs Institute in Australia as a response to the need to develop a method for the analysis and synthesis of qualitative research that cannot be analysed within a meta-analysis. In the Reviewers' Manual for the Joanna Briggs Institute, meta-aggregation is described as a method that mirrors the process of a quantitative review, while holding onto the traditions and requirements of qualitative research.

In a meta-aggregative review, papers are searched for according to clear inclusion and exclusion criteria and critically appraised. Data analysis and synthesis involves the aggregation of evidence using themes rather than statistics, and the aim of the review is a summary of the themes identified in the papers included in the review. Meta-aggregative reviews are described as the assembly and combination of many research findings into a whole that is more than the sum of the individual parts.

The meta-aggregative approach is described as one that emphasizes the complexities of the research while providing a synthesis that is transparent and that results in synthesized statements which are practical and usable (Hannes and Lockwood 2011), an attribute that, it is argued, makes this approach attractive to policy-makers and practitioners. Indeed, Hannes and Lockwood (2011) refer to meta-aggregation as a pragmatic approach, citing the work of John Dewey (1938) and his understanding of pragmatism as: 'the meaning … of any thought or idea [is] determined by criteria of practical usefulness' (2011: 1636).

Example of a systematic review with meta-aggregation

Sun and colleagues (2025) used the methods of meta-aggregation described by the Joanna Briggs Institute (Hannes and Lockwood 2011) to compile evidence on the impact of the COVID-19 pandemic on working conditions and nursing practices in acute care hospital environments including intensive care units and emergency departments. The authors selected qualitative research which they combined using meta-aggregation to identify eight categories which they defined as unfavourable working conditions or harmful to nursing staff. The implications for this type of review might be helpful to nurse managers faced with future pandemics or health crises.

When might a meta-aggregative review be appropriate for your post-graduate study?

For anyone considering a meta-aggregative approach to their literature review, Hannes and Lockwood (2011) argue that concepts need to be well developed rather than exploratory and in the analysis researchers should be aiming for a clear and transparent relationship between the participants' experience and the related themes (2011: 1636). This is because the aim of meta-aggregation is to summarize rather than to interpret, and to achieve a pragmatic and reliable representation of the themes arising in the literature.

For example, Grover et al. (2023) undertook a meta-aggregative systematic review using a Joanna Briggs Institute approach to investigate social prescribing for older adults. Social prescribing is a complex intervention that seeks to foster networks of community support and may help to mitigate loneliness in older people (those over 60 years). The authors searched for qualitative and mixed-methods research designs. Despite limited evidence they drew out findings for primary care providers. The meta-aggregative approach can be regarded as the qualitative equivalent to a meta-analysis. The results of the studies are pooled together so that the findings of ten studies are stronger than the findings of one study.

Focused mapping review and synthesis

This is an approach to mapping the trends in publication of literature in your area. Similar to a scoping study, the focused mapping review and synthesis is designed to describe and quantify trends in terms or concepts used in published papers. It can also demonstrate which treatments and interventions come into and go out of fashion. For example, it enables the reviewer to determine what research methodologies are popular in the published literature, which journals they are published in and the countries from which the research is published. The focused mapping review and synthesis does not incorporate all the steps of a formal literature review and does not include critical appraisal or detailed analysis and synthesis of the literature, but is an approach used to map volume and trends in the published literature on a particular topic.

Example of a focused mapping review and synthesis

Aveyard and Bradbury-Jones (2019) undertook a focused mapping review and synthesis to explore the trends in the publication of literature reviews in five highly ranked nursing journals. This approach enabled the authors to determine which approaches to doing a literature review were most used and how they were undertaken, highlighting patterns and inconsistencies in the publication of literature reviews.

When might a focused mapping review and synthesis be appropriate for your post-graduate study?

You may consider using a focused mapping review and synthesis as a component of your literature review in a doctoral or PhD study where you have the opportunity to explore many different methodological aspects of your study (we will discuss this in Chapter 3), and an examination of the publication and methodological trends in your research area can help you to set the context for your study. For example, Mills et al. (2024) undertook this approach in order to explore the frequency and content of papers published with the following terms (which are often used interchangeably): shared decision-making – patient participation in decision-making – informed consent. This enabled the author team to identify the frequency of use of each term as evidenced by publications and how the terms are used in contemporary literature.

Qualitative evidence synthesis

For anyone undertaking a literature review in which their aim is not to summarize but to interpret, there are methods that facilitate the further interpretation of the data. Some methods are specific to the analysis of qualitative methods and some can be used with mixed methods. In this section, we focus on the synthesis of qualitative methods.

Meta-ethnography was developed by Noblit and Hare (1988) as an alternative to the pragmatic summary and aggregation of themes identified in a review. Meta-ethnography was one of the first documented approaches to the analysis of qualitative research and represents a move away from meta-aggregation. The aim of a meta-ethnography is not the combination of the results of qualitative data but the search for new interpretations from the data. The features involved in a meta-ethnography are similar to those described previously, but in the analysis there is a focus on interpretation, rather than on providing a simple summary of the data. For those of you undertaking an interpretive analysis, the results are:

> *integrations that are more than the sum of the parts, in that they offer novel interpretations of findings. These interpretations will not be found in any one research report but rather are inferences derived from taking all of the reports in a sample as a whole.*
>
> (Thorne et al. 2004: 1358)

Despite the name given to this method and the initial focus on the interpretation of ethnographic studies, the authors advised that their approach was not limited to the analysis and synthesis of ethnographic studies and could be used far more extensively to analyse a wide range of qualitative research studies. However, a meta-ethnography does not include quantitative studies.

In order to emphasize the inclusivity of this interpretive approach, further adaptations of meta-ethnography were developed: **meta-interpretation** (Finfgeld 1999), **thematic synthesis** (Thomas and Harden 2008) and **meta-synthesis** (Stern and Harris 1985; Walsh and Downe 2005). These approaches share the common features of a literature review as described on page 3 but they emphasize that all qualitative studies can be included, rather than just ethnographic studies. These approaches are based on the original work of Noblit and Hare (1988).

Example of a systematic review with an interpretive approach

Bartoli et al. (2025) undertook a meta-synthesis to investigate the factors involved in the transition from hospital to home of stroke patients, including the training and support needs of the people with stroke, their families and healthcare providers. While people who have a stroke are initially treated in hospital, they will need to continue their recovery at home, despite 75 per cent having long-term disabilities. In this study, the authors did more than report the different studies; they compared and contrasted the differences between the studies using a critical-interpretive approach to their meta-synthesis.

When might an interpretive approach for the review of qualitative studies be appropriate for your post-graduate study?

Although Noblit and Hare (1988) argue that the meta-ethnographic approach is not for the novice, this interpretive approach might be appropriate when you aim to explore and interpret concepts in detail rather than simply report and summarize the findings of a range of studies. They are useful when the concepts explored in a review are difficult to define and require further clarification within the review. An interpretive approach can only be used with qualitative studies.

For example, Fernández-Basanta et al. (2020) undertook a meta-ethnography to explore coping strategies of parents in different cultures following perinatal loss. We contacted the authors of this study. In an email correspondence, Sara Fernández-Basanta (2020) described why they undertook a meta-ethnography for this study:

> *We selected the meta-ethnography methodology because it allows condensing the qualitative knowledge of a specific area of interest, and therefore generating results that promote evidence-based care. This methodology combines results interpretively rather than in an aggregative way, providing a deeper and broader understanding than the results of individual studies. Its objective is not to synthesize the truth but to search for different perspectives within and between studies. Our qualitative review was carried out following the approach proposed by Noblit and Hare (1988), who developed this methodology.*

4 Integrative reviews

In this section, we focus on the integration and re-interpretation of a variety of research (and sometimes non-research) methods. Despite initial concern about combining qualitative and quantitative research in a literature review due to different methodological considerations (Jensen and Allen 1996; Rogers et al. 1996), there has been increasing recognition that research from a diverse range of research methods may be relevant to a particular research question and could be – and indeed should be – examined within one literature review.

Harden and Thomas (2005) argue that research questions should not be confined in their answers by the type of study but by relevance of the study to the research question, and hence should incorporate a range of study designs in their reviews. Thus, recent developments have seen approaches that advocate the combination of different types of research and other evidence, including theoretical evidence.

The integrative review is an approach that incorporates the integration of a wide range of literature in a review rather than just qualitative methods and was developed by Whittemore and Knafl (2005). The integrative review is described by them as:

> *the broadest type of research review methods, allowing for the simultaneous inclusion of experimental and non experimental research in order to more fully understand a phenomena of concern …*

> *Integrative reviewers may also combine data from the theoretical as well as empirical literature.*
>
> (Whittemore and Knafl 2005: 547)

The questions defined by someone undertaking an integrative review can be broad, the aim of which may be to define concepts, review theories or analyse methodological issues. A diverse range of literature can therefore be included in an integrative review. The integrative review outlines the features of a literature review as presented on page 3. A well-defined question is followed by a comprehensive search, then data extraction and critical appraisal. In data analysis, data are coded, ordered and categorized. Whittemore and Knafl argue that '[a] thorough and unbiased interpretation of primary sources along with an innovative synthesis of the evidence, are the goals of the data analysis stage' (2005: 550). The aim of the analysis is the thorough and unbiased interpretation of primary sources, along with an innovative synthesis. The integrative review can be used to define concepts, review theories and analyse methods (Whittemore and Knafl 2005), in addition to the analysis of empirical research to address a clinically relevant question (Flemming 2010; Niela-Vilén et al. 2014).

The **mixed-methods review** is a similar approach to an integrative review but focuses on the combination of qualitative and quantitative research in the review in order to provide a broader picture of the existing research but does not widen its approach to include non-research data. This approach is described by Lizarondo et al. (2024) and is available online via the JBI Reviewers Manual.

Example of a mixed-methods review

Bench et al. (2021) undertook a mixed-methods review of the experience of survivors of critical illness. The authors combined studies from different research methods in order to utilize the broad range of research on the topic that did not reflect any one research method. The majority of studies were quantitative and identified the prevalence of fatigue as the overriding finding. The authors recommended that further qualitative research should be undertaken in order to understand this experience further.

When might an interpretive approach to a review of the mix of qualitative and quantitative studies be appropriate for your post-graduate study?

A mixed-methods approach to your literature review might be appropriate when you have a combination of research designs that are relevant to your research question rather than literature that fits into either a 'quantitative' or 'qualitative' design category. For example, Qian et al. (2025) undertook a mixed-methods integrative review to identify barriers to recognizing and treating delirium in people being cared for in specialist palliative care contexts. They used a convergent-integrated Joanna Briggs Institute approach to data synthesis.

5 Paradigm or theory-driven reviews

These reviews focus on the development of theory and can include some of the approaches used in the reviews described above, thus illustrating the complexity of categorizing methods for doing a literature review. Furthermore, some of these approaches might also be categorized as qualitative evidence synthesis or mixed-methods reviews.

Critical interpretive synthesis was developed by Dixon-Woods et al. (2006) and is closely based on meta-ethnography and the work of Noblit and Hare (1988) with reference to grounded theory. The authors emphasize that the method can be used with a wide range of research and other evidence and hence can be more broadly applied than a meta-ethnography. Critical interpretive synthesis is therefore another approach that incorporates a wide range of literature in an interpretive review. The aim of critical interpretive synthesis is the generation of a theory and the developments of new concepts, so it is a more focused approach than the integrative review but in many ways could be included in the section above, illustrating the difficulties in achieving a clear classification of approaches to doing a review. The methods involved in critical interpretive synthesis reflect those used in a grounded theory, for example the inductive forming of the review question and theoretical sampling for included literature. Dixon-Woods et al. (2006) describe how, in their qualitative review of the literature, they initially set out to use a meta-ethnographic approach but found that it did not seem suitable for their study of a large number of disparate studies, including quantitative studies. As a result, the researchers adapted the meta-ethnography technique to one that incorporated the use of a wide range of studies but that retained the essence of constant comparative analysis and interpretation. This also facilitated the development of theory. Dixon-Woods et al. (2006) argue that since the generation of theory is often based on a broad range of evidence, not just empirical research studies, non-research evidence should be included in the synthesis if appropriate. Like Noblit and Hare, they focus on the identification of a purposive sample rather than a comprehensive sample of literature.

Narrative synthesis is defined as a form of storytelling, relying on words and text to summarize and explain the data in a literature review (Popay et al. 2006; Pope et al. 2007). The method was developed as a response to the need to formalize systematic review methods that were not associated with a meta-analysis as described earlier. Popay et al. (2006: 11) describe four elements to a narrative synthesis, although they emphasize that these need not be undertaken in a linear way:

1. Developing a theory of how the intervention works, why and for whom
2. Developing a preliminary synthesis of findings of included studies
3. Exploring relationships in the data
4. Assessing the robustness of the synthesis.

Hence, although the primary aim of narrative synthesis is to develop an understanding of the empirical studies, it is also an approach that emphasizes the role of theory. People undertaking a narrative synthesis often commence their review with the identification of relevant theories that underpin the question they are reviewing. After defining a research review question, the reviewers follow the features of a literature review identified earlier. The narrative synthesis approach described by Popay et al. (2006) offers a wide variety of methods for the analysis and synthesis of literature including descriptions, tabulating data, content analysis, thematic analysis, concept and ideas mapping, and qualitative case descriptions for the development of theory.

When might a narrative synthesis be appropriate for your post-graduate study?

A narrative synthesis might be appropriate for your review when you have a combination of research designs and where you are interested in exploring these in relation to established theories and concepts.

For example, Dunleavy et al. (2018) undertook a narrative synthesis to explore barriers and facilitators to the recruitment of patients and carers within palliative care. In an email correspondence, Lesley Dunleavy (2025) explained the rationale for using a narrative synthesis approach to their review:

> *A narrative synthesis review was chosen as it became apparent during initial searches of the literature that it was important to be able to include non-research as well as primary research data to*

answer the review question. The evidence available was more likely to be authors reflecting on and writing about their observations of the palliative care trial recruitment process rather than primary research data. These observations help us to understand what the barriers and facilitators are to patient and carer recruitment in palliative care randomized controlled trials. Popay et al.'s (2006) narrative synthesis framework was used to guide the literature review process as it facilitates the inclusion of research and non-research data and the use of theory to inform the data extraction and interpretation process.

The meta-narrative is a method that incorporates the integration of a wide range of literature and emphasizes the importance of the theoretical background of the studies within the review. The meta-narrative approach was developed by Greenhalgh et al. (2005) and Pope and Mays (2006), and further described by Wong et al. (2013b), who describe how a topic or phenomenon might have been examined in a variety of different ways, using different philosophical approaches, all of which might contribute to an enhanced understanding. Meta-narrative reviews draw on the work of Kuhn (1962), who argued that scientific paradigms evolve over time and research should be considered within the paradigm within which it was conducted. A meta-narrative review explores the paradigm in addition to the research that has been identified as relevant to the review. In order to incorporate research from different research traditions, in a meta-narrative approach, research is compared initially from within its own paradigm so that any inconsistencies within the data can be explored within the paradigm in which it was generated.

When might a meta-narrative review be appropriate for your post-graduate study?

A meta-narrative review is concerned with the exploration of research within the paradigm in which it is undertaken. In an email correspondence, Laurel Mimmo (2020) explained why her team used a meta-narrative approach for their study (Mimmo et al. 2019):

Stemming from our previous work, we wanted to explore parental experiences of care when their child with intellectual disability was admitted to hospital. Following the PRISMA guidelines we conducted a systematic review of the literature, and during the initial searches of the literature we found that the limited number of studies that fitted our inclusion criteria had comparable findings whilst coming from disparate health research disciplines. On discussion with my supervisor we determined that a meta-narrative approach, that incorporated consideration of the methods by which the study was undertaken in addition to the results themselves, was the most appropriate way to synthesise and report the findings.

The realist review is an approach to reviewing literature that is grounded in a realist philosophy of science (Bhaskar 1978). The purpose of a realist review is to explore why a programme or intervention works, in what circumstances and for whom, rather than just to ask the question 'does it work?' (Pawson et al. 2005; Jagosh 2019). The aim is explanation and in particular the review and development of theories that underlie an intervention. It draws on the same principles as a realist evaluation (Pawson and Tilley 1997), and a realist review can be used in conjunction with or independently of an empirical realist evaluation. On this basis, realist reviews often use the Context + Mechanism = Outcome configuration (CMOc) to guide data synthesis.

Realist reviews allow researchers to focus on the phenomenon of interest, and explore possible relationships between context, programme design, implementation, mechanisms and outcomes. Realist reviews have the advantage over other review methods in that they allow for detailed consideration of a broad and complex intervention. They take into account the fact that, for example, paediatric palliative care services require the active input of individuals, specialists and non-specialists, who are embedded in social infrastructures such as hospitals and community services, and whose roles are influenced by others, including patients and colleagues. The impact of institutional and system factors, such as local and national policy guidance and commissioning, provide further complexity (Mitchell et al. 2020).

A realist review has some things in common with other literature review approaches, but also possesses critical differences. The search for underlying theory is a central component of its search strategy. Subsequently, realist reviewers articulate candidate theories (e.g. a middle range or programme theory) to be explored alongside their review question. Developing and refining theory will often require an iterative literature search approach that may involve multiple cycles of interrogating studies and then conducting more searches based on emergent theories or areas of interest. Studies and data should be appraised in light of the usefulness of their evidence. This means that pre-existing critical appraisal tools may not be appropriate. Realist reviews allow diverse studies to be included, which may include studies involving different populations or conceptually similar programmes, because the focus of interest is on extracting relevant information – evidence 'nuggets' – that are pertinent to the review question.

Example of a realist review

Harris et al. (2019) conducted a realist review for their work on diabetes research, In an email correspondence, Janet Harris (2020) wrote the following: '*We decided to do a realist review exploring whether patient and community involvement in diabetes research influences health outcomes, for several reasons. In terms of background knowledge, there were a number of emerging strands of literature indicating that when people are actively involved in their own treatment plans, they may experience more success in self managing their chronic and long term conditions. In the field of participatory research, models were also emerging that indicated that participation in co-designing services and support can contribute to a sense of empowerment, increased well being and increased agency. At the same time, systematic reviews of the effectiveness of diabetes interventions in promoting self management and improving health outcomes were equivocal. This led us to wonder whether the process of involvement may be an "active ingredient", that might have an undocumented influence on ability to manage diabetes. Consultations with diabetes practitioners indicated that from their perspective, engagement was key in self-management. A scoping search revealed a set of papers that appeared to use involvement and participation when designing and implementing diabetes interventions; albeit in diverse ways. From a reviewer perspective, we could have decided at this point to simply limit ourselves to an effectiveness review. This direction, however, would have excluded studies that contained rich descriptions of the phenomenon of interest - which was participation and involvement. Conversely, going in the direction of a qualitative evidence synthesis also presented limitations. If health outcome studies were excluded, we would not have been able to explore whether there were any relationships between involvement and ability to self manage diabetes. A realist review therefore seemed the best approach, for several reasons*'.

When might a realist review be appropriate for your post-graduate study?

A realist review is likely to be used by someone interested in the context and paradigm in which the study is located and the influence of this on the findings or results of the study. A realistic review is focused on an understanding of how, why, for whom and in what circumstances an intervention works. It is a complex method and should ideally be undertaken by a group of researchers. For example, Lyman et al. (2019) undertook a realist review to explore organizational learning in hospitals in order to develop middle range theory. In an email correspondence, Bret Lyman (2020) explained why they undertook a realist review:

> *We selected a realist approach for our review because we wanted to develop a pragmatic theory about a complex, context-dependent phenomenon [organizational learning]. From the beginning of our inquiry, we recognized it would be folly to presume that any single evidence-based intervention could be effective in every situation. Rather, we felt it would be more meaningful to address the question, 'What works, for whom, in what circumstances, and why?' (Rycroft-Malone et al., 2012, p. 3). Our objective was well served by the inclusive nature of realist inquiry, which allowed us to consider information from a wide variety of sources and did not restrict our inquiry to a finite number of potential factors. We used the Realist And MEta-narrative Evidence Syntheses: Evolving Standards (RAMESES) publication standards (Wong et al., 2013[a]) to guide our inquiry.*

6 Overview of reviews

Some literature reviews are designed to provide an overview of literature in an area. An overview of reviews or 'umbrella' review is a term used for a literature review of existing literature reviews. As more reviews are published, reviewing these reviews is becoming an essential task so that we can understand the summary of existing reviews. The term 'umbrella review' was coined by the JBI Institute and the methodology was developed by Aromataris et al. (2014). A clear description of the method is also provided by Choi and Kang (2023). If, for example, the search on the topic you are interested in identifies many pre-existing reviews, in order to find out the existing knowledge in the area, instead of identifying all the original papers, a more pragmatic approach would be to review the existing reviews. Umbrella reviews are therefore a useful method for synthesizing the ever-expanding volume of reviews.

Brenan et al. (2020) undertook an umbrella review to explore nursing handovers. In an email correspondence, one of the authors, Alvisa Palese (2020) explained:

After a first check of the literature, we have discovered that in recent years several systematic reviews were conducted and published in the field of nursing handovers. However, it emerged also that no attempts were conducted to summarize the several reviews available in a single, accessible evidence-based report. As a result, we were in front of several reviews with a clear perception of a fragmented knowledge. We reflected about the potential consequences of this fragmentation on nurses, managers, policy makers, educators and researchers in their need to have a comprehensive understanding of the evidence available on nursing handovers which might tremendously affect patients' safety. Therefore, we have undertaken an umbrella review methodology with the intent to:

- *detect, extract, assess and organize a wide range of review-level evidence published in the field;*
- *summarize what was known about nursing handovers and to synthesize the evidence into one practical document, useful for clinical nurses, nurse managers, educators and policy-makers, by reporting what is known and highlighting recommendations for practice;*
- *identify a potential lack of knowledge, uncertainties and research gaps aimed at highlighting recommendations to support researchers to better understand and evaluate the directions in the research field.*

When might an umbrella review be appropriate for your post-graduate study?

We suggest that the need for an umbrella review usually indicates that the research topic in question is too large for doctoral-level study, however it might illustrate an important aspect of the background for your study. It is an important method to be aware of, and an understanding of the process of doing an umbrella review will be useful to you, even if you do not undertake the method in its entirety.

In summary

There are many approaches to reviewing the literature and we have not attempted to present all of them in this chapter; methods of literature reviewing are continuously being developed and refined, and any attempt to present a comprehensive overview would be quickly out of date. The methods we have presented are illustrative of the different types of approaches that are available.

While it is not necessary to follow a specified approach to your literature review within your post-graduate project, it is recommended that you consider all the common features of a review, which we outline on page 3. Most reviews share the common features of a research question, searching strategy, then appraisal of the research or other evidence identified, which leads to a summary or interpretation of the results. Depending on the type of review you undertake, you will find that a different emphasis is placed on different features – for example, some reviews set clear criteria for quality assessment and do not include studies that do not meet those criteria, while others are more inclusive. These features are discussed throughout the book and it is important that you can justify the approach you undertake for your review.

If you do follow a specific approach to a literature review, we recommend that you access the relevant texts that describe this approach in full detail. As with all research methods, innovations and new ideas about possible methods are regularly published in academic journals and should be accessed if you decide to follow a particular approach.

The approach you take to your literature review will largely depend on the aim of your review and the type of research and other evidence that is relevant to it, as outlined in Table 2.1. Some literature reviews can be undertaken in a highly controlled way so that potential factors that might bias the outcomes are reduced and the review aims to provide a numerical (statistical) summary of the results, such as a systematic review with meta-analysis. Other literature reviews do not aim to summarize the findings numerically but seek to describe and interpret the findings in order to provide a textual (thematic) summary of the results. Other approaches aim to incorporate both a numerical and thematic summary of the findings.

You will note that we have not included rapid reviews in this categorization. As their name implies, rapid reviews are undertaken within a specific timeframe, often due to funding or other constraints for which expediency requires a more immediate project and a corresponding reduction in the depth or detail needed in a review. For students studying at post-graduate level, this is unlikely to be the case and hence we have not included this approach in this chapter.

Key points

- The methods for reviewing the literature have recently become more explicit and rigorous and are continuously being developed
- You may decide to follow an explicit method for your review
- All methods share common features, which should be evident in all reviews
- There are also some significant differences between the methods described
- You need to be able to justify the approach you have taken when you write up your project or defend it in an oral examination.

3

What research and other evidence should I include in my literature review?

In this chapter, we will discuss:

- *How empirical research will be relevant to your review*
- *How theories and concepts will be relevant to your review*
- *How research methods will be relevant to your review.*

In Chapter 2, we discussed the different methods that have been developed for undertaking a literature review. In this chapter, we will discuss the research and other evidence that you may include in your review. There is so much published information that you need to be able to recognize what is – and what is not – relevant for answering your review question. This will be guided by your research question, and your inclusion and exclusion criteria.

There are different types of literature that you are likely to engage with at different times in your review. When you are contemplating a literature review, it is often a review of the empirical research literature that you may think of initially, and indeed the empirical review is usually the main focus of a review of the literature. By empirical literature we mean both qualitative and quantitative research, in addition to mixed-methods research, in which data has been collected using observational or experimental methods, providing evidence about what has already been observed or known about the area you are studying. This is because, in many cases, an empirical literature review will underpin a forthcoming empirical study or, for a standalone literature review, empirical literature is often best suited to answering your research question. However, this is not always the case and it depends on your question and the inclusion and exclusion criteria you set.

In a detailed research project, you are also likely to include a section in which you discuss the research methods used in the papers you have identified in order to help you select and defend your choice of methods and to understand the research methods used by others. You are also likely to consider the underlying theories and concepts in the papers you use in order to fully understand the background to the papers you use and to help provide an explanatory framework with which to interpret the literature you include in your review.

For this reason, your review might have different sections in which you discuss different types of literature that build up the argument for a project. These are often empirical, theoretical and methodological; though not necessarily all three. The structure will depend on the needs of your project. If your review is divided into different sections, each will have its own focus and its own review question, and the literature you include within each section will depend on the literature review question and the inclusion and exclusion criteria you identify.

- The *empirical* literature is important as this enables you to bring together all the empirical research studies that have been undertaken which fit your inclusion and exclusion criteria.
- The *theoretical* literature is important in your review to ensure that your work, and the work of others, is understood and set within an appropriate theoretical framework. The data provided by your empirical literature review or your subsequent empirical study needs to be set in the context of other theories in order to make sense of and explain the results that you have.
- The *methodological* literature is important to your review as you are likely to refer to research undertaken in similar areas in order to help you to plan and justify the approaches you use in your own study. You also need to be able to understand the strengths and limitations of the methods used by others whose work you include in your review.

Given the large amount of information you are likely to come across, it can be difficult to know where to start. Wallace and Wray (2021) present a system for categorizing evidence and identify four different types: theory, research, practice and policy. This can be useful as it will prompt you to consider the information you have against these categories and hence whether it is relevant to your review. Given the diversity of health and social care information, this assignment may not always be a straightforward task.

In general terms, in our experience, Wallace and Wray's (2021) categories of theory and research are likely to be the types of literature most important to you in your review. This is because many review questions tend to be answered by data obtained from the systematic observation or experiments from the practice environment in health and social care, and the associated concepts and theories. In contrast, practice literature refers to discussion and accounts of practice and may not be assessed as rigorous evidence for inclusion in the results section of your review but may provide useful background information. Similarly, policies and guidelines are generally derived from research but in themselves may not constitute rigorous evidence for inclusion within a review. However, there is a caveat here; if your literature review question requires the review of policies or informal discussion or opinion, you would, of course, include this literature in your review.

If you are doing a larger empirical project such as a PhD or doctorate, you will need to think carefully about what aspects of the literature you need to consider in detail before you commence your own empirical work. The detail in which you are able to review the literature will depend on the scope of your study; it is particularly important if you are studying for a professional or taught doctorate or PhD but is also relevant to a research project that is a component of a MSc or master's award or a smaller-scale study.

Identifying different types of evidence you will draw on in your review

Forde-Johnson (2020) undertook a PhD study looking at the use of electronic patient records (EPR) and the way that this affects nurse-patient communication and the development of a therapeutic relationship. A tool that has been developed to measure nurse-patient communication was adapted for use in this study. In order to provide a robust justification for the study, Forde-Johnson identified two possible areas for which thorough review of the literature was considered essential: first, a review of empirical studies that have explored the effect of electronic means of recording care on the nurse-patient relationship and, second, a review of the development, use and adaptation of an existing tool for measuring communication, or in other words a review of *methods* for measuring nurse-patient communication. The first review of empirical research that explored the effect of electronic records on nurse-patient communication was published (Ford-Johnson et al. 2023). The second review of the development of the tool was unpublished but was a key component of the thesis. We use this example to illustrate how your project might require different reviews to set the background context for your study. This might require careful identification and you might not anticipate that more than one review is needed when you embark on a study.

Empirical literature

Empirical research literature refers to studies where researchers use direct observation or experience to attempt to answer a research question. Sometimes the observations and experiences are collected in the natural environment and sometimes they are manipulated, as in an experiment, for example. Data about observations and experience can be collected either qualitatively using textual descriptions or quantitatively using numerical measures, or sometimes using mixed methods where a combination of both qualitative and quantitative approaches is used. Both qualitative and quantitative data can be analysed thematically. Quantitative data can sometimes be analysed statistically.

There is a broad range of empirical research designs, from classic experiments (often referred to as randomized controlled trials, or RCTs) to variations on the classical experiment (for example, cluster RCTs or quasi-experiments), to surveys, and there is a wide variety of qualitative approaches. Empirical research is often discussed in terms of the paradigm from which it is associated. For example, quantitative approaches are often aligned to a positivist paradigm and qualitative approaches to an interpretivist paradigm. There is no one approach to empirical study that is 'better' than another but some are more suited to answering certain questions than others. Quantitative approaches are ideal for measuring that which is easily measurable and where direct comparisons are possible. Qualitative approaches are ideal for answering questions that seek in-depth meaning about a topic, or where an exploratory approach is required. Qualitative approaches are often undertaken where little is already known, and quantitative approaches are ideal for looking at relationships between concepts that are already well defined.

It is beyond the scope of this book to discuss the paradigm debates or to explore all the major empirical methods but we strongly recommend that you are familiar with these methods before you commence your post-graduate studies. A research methods textbook should help facilitate this.

Grey literature

Grey literature refers to unpublished work such as a dissertation or other unpublished report. Grey literature is not published in a traditional format and is not easily accessed by electronic databases; however, there are some databases specific to the retrieval of grey literature. Non-academic journals might be referred to as grey literature and other information such as hospital policies also fall into this category. The inclusion of grey literature within your post-graduate thesis requires some thought and discussion with your supervisor. Inclusion of literature that has not been formally published and therefore not subject to the peer review process might lead you to including poorer-quality literature. On the other hand, the exclusion of unpublished literature might lead to the exclusion of practical experiences and accounts from patients. For these reasons, you need to consider carefully how and if you will include grey literature.

Inclusion of empirical literature in your literature review

The empirical literature that you include in your review will depend on the research question you are asking, but there are subtle differences in what you include depending on whether your review supports a larger study or is a standalone study in its own right.

- When the literature review is supportive and a prerequisite to a larger empirical study, the empirical literature will generally be used to determine what has been done before and to identify the gap in the knowledge that will shape the research question for the larger study. Hence, the aim of the review is to demonstrate the need and rationale for your subsequent empirical study.
- When the literature review is a standalone review, the empirical literature will generally be used to answer – or attempt to answer – the

research question. Hence, the aim of the review is to demonstrate what we know, rather than to demonstrate a gap in knowledge. However, this difference can be subtle as a standalone review can demonstrate that there is insufficient evidence to answer the review question.

The important point is that you recognize the role of the literature review and what it is helping you to achieve within your project.

Which empirical evidence is best for my literature review?

Some empirical studies will be better suited to addressing your literature review question than others. It is important that you can make a judgement about what studies will be most useful in answering your research question. There are practical and academic reasons to do this. Practically, there is a lot of published information for almost every research question. Identifying the most appropriate evidence to include in your review is an important consideration so that you do not have to wade through a lot of inappropriate literature. Academically, given that certain types of empirical research are going to be more relevant than others, it is important to identify what these are so that your search for relevant empirical research is focused.

Different types of study designs are useful for answering different questions. Although RCTs are often used by Cochrane Collaboration reviewers, these reviews are usually focused on answering questions about effectiveness and so these studies are appropriate. Even so, only RCTs that include sufficient information to calculate effect sizes can be included. For other literature review questions, other study designs are likely to be more relevant, and the type of study design that is most relevant will be determined by the literature review in question as we discussed in Chapters 1 and 2.

It can therefore be useful to identify the types of study designs that are most likely to inform your literature review, so that you can search for these in the first instance. While prior identification of possible relevant study designs will not be definitive, it will help to guide you to what is likely to be appropriate for inclusion in your literature review in the first instance.

Considerations of hierarchies of evidence

You may come across the term 'hierarchy of evidence'. This term refers to the positivist tradition of ranking research and other evidence in terms of research designs which are most likely to eliminate bias. Bias is eliminated using strategies such as randomization and blinding, and those studies which are able to control for this are considered to be the least biased. Hierarchies of evidence are based on the principle that certain types of research designs will be less biased than others.

The most well-known hierarchy of evidence was developed by Sackett et al. (1996) in order to rank which research designs provide the strongest evidence for determining the effectiveness of a treatment or intervention. This hierarchy is based on the assumption that studies that provide a direct comparison of a treatment or intervention are the best way to determine effectiveness, that controlling for bias within studies is possible and that studies with the least bias will provide the strongest evidence. This hierarchy places systematic review of RCTs at the top, followed by RCTs, and qualitative studies near the bottom, because of the ability of RCTs to determine the effectiveness of treatments and interventions due to the rigour and degree of control that they have (Figure 3.1).

This hierarchy of evidence is well known but it can be misleading when doing a literature review. While systematic reviews of RCTs include highly controlled studies that aim to eliminate bias as far as is possible, they may not be relevant to answering your literature review question. The hierarchy is *only* relevant for literature review questions that are concerned with measuring the effectiveness of interventions.

1. Evidence from systematic reviews of RCTs	↑	**Highest**
2. Evidence from RCTs		
3. Evidence from cohort studies, case-controlled studies		
4. Evidence from surveys		
5. Evidence in the form of case reports		
6. Evidence in the form of qualitative studies		
7. Evidence from experts	↓	
8. Anecdotal opinion		**Lowest**

Figure 3.1 Hierarchy of evidence for determining the effectiveness of a treatment or intervention

Despite this, the hierarchy developed by Sackett et al. (1996) is sometimes over-simplified and referred to as 'the hierarchy of evidence' (Hoppe et al. 2009), implying that RCTs are always stronger than other studies in terms of the strength of evidence they provide. Given that different review questions will be best informed by different study designs, clearly there is no one 'hierarchy of evidence' that can be applied indiscriminately to all literature review questions; nor is there one type of research design that is always the most relevant to all literature review questions (as discussed in the early chapters of this book).

Identifying which empirical research will be relevant for your review

To start at the beginning, if your literature review question addresses an exploratory question about which little is known, you may seek other exploratory studies to help address the question. Qualitative studies are likely to be useful in this instance. If, on the other hand, your literature review addresses a question about the relationship between different concepts that can be directly compared, then the literature that you include is likely to be that which has already analysed these relationships. Quantitative studies may be useful here. It is important to note that your final literature review is likely to include a broader range of literature than this brief summary might indicate, but it can be helpful to consider which literature you will be looking for in the first instance, to get your literature review underway.

Before you undertake your empirical literature review, you should write a protocol or plan for your study. This will enable you to identify the literature that is relevant for your review. For example, researchers whose protocol for a systematic review is registered with the Cochrane Collaboration will consider and plan the type of literature they will seek in addressing their review question. If the question concerns the effectiveness of an intervention (for example, Cochrane systematic reviews with meta-analysis), reviewers are likely to indicate that they will be looking for RCTs – or reviews of RCTs – in the first instance, if these are available.

However, if your literature review question is investigating how social workers approach conversations about confidentiality in their practice, you would probably need to include a number of different research designs, and RCTs would probably not be relevant. In this case, you would be looking for research that explores the practice of social workers in a day-to-day context. This might include a range of qualitative and observational research designs from case studies involving interviews with practitioners and also interviews with their clients.

If you are exploring the impact of introducing smoke-free policies in a setting, you would be searching for literature that explores the views and attitudes and actions of people who live or work within that setting. This literature is likely to consist of exploratory interviews, focus groups and possibly questionnaires, in addition to before-and-after studies that explore changes in rates of smoking.

So you can see that there is no one type of research design that is most appropriate for the different literature review questions mentioned above. The type of research design you need to include depends entirely on your research question.

Finding the appropriate evidence for your study

Given that different literature review questions require different research designs to answer them, in 2010 Noyes identified alternative 'hierarchies' that may be appropriate for different literature review questions. Noyes (2010) argued that qualitative approaches can be used to answer more exploratory questions, such as when exploring patients' or clients' views and experiences of services and interventions. She emphasized that, in this case, qualitative studies are likely to be more useful for describing patient or client experiences than quantitative studies, and this will be reflected in the literature identified in the search for relevant research. Noyes (2010: 530) gave an example of a hierarchy of evidence that could help us understand client or patient experience. The hierarchy of 'views and experiences of interventions and services' is given in Figure 3.2.

Qualitative studies can also be used to examine many types of research question, such as why people behave in a certain way, what the needs of a group of people are, whether a treatment or intervention is feasible, whether a treatment or intervention can be improved, and so on. Hierarchies of evidence can be a useful way to begin to consider which research methods are most relevant to your research question. However, they are a guide only and need to be considered flexibly – otherwise you risk omitting relevant literature from your review. Some researchers would express caution at the concept of any attempt to rank evidence, and would argue that it is problematic and over-simplistic and fails to engage with the complexities of the research you might come across. For example, these hierarchies place an order for certain studies but do not take into account how you should consider a study that is placed high in a hierarchy and is relevant to the review question but that has methodological flaws that affect its design and conduct.

1. Evidence from systematic reviews of well-designed qualitative studies	▲	**Highest**
2. Evidence from systematic reviews of mixed-methods approaches	│	
3. Evidence from one well-conducted qualitative study	│	
4. Evidence from well-designed research and consumer surveys	│	
5. Evidence in the form of opinion of lay people	│	
6. Evidence in the form of quantitative studies	▼	**Lowest**

Figure 3.2 Hierarchy of evidence for understanding the views and experiences of services users

Despite the complexities in the arguments, some research designs will be better suited to answering your review question than others, and it is important to identify this when planning your literature review. Having a predetermined idea of the type of research designs that you might include to answer your literature review question can be a useful way to commence your literature review, even if, on further engagement with the literature, you adapt and change your view of what research designs are most useful in answering your question.

Using empirical literature to justify your research question

When your literature review is a prerequisite to a larger study, the empirical literature review is usually where you justify your research question. By reviewing the existing studies, the gap in knowledge becomes evident. The following example from Forde-Johnson et al. (2023) illustrates this process.

Developing your research question

The use of electronic records is widely prevalent in the majority of healthcare facilities. They provide a practical and permanent record of patient care which has clear and obvious benefits for staff and patients alike. A PhD student and senior nurse, Forde-Johnson was aware of a potential downside however. Clinical nurses in her team reported an overt reliance on technology, which affected the way they interacted with their patients. Using this anecdotal evidence as a trigger for further enquiry, Forde-Johnson developed a proposal to explore the effect of electronic records on communication and interaction between nurses and their patients. The first task was to review the empirical evidence already published to find out what is known about the effect of electronic records on nurse-patient interaction and communication. The focus of published work was on GP and primary healthcare consultations identifying a clear gap to explore interactions within a hospital setting (Forde-Johnson et al. 2023).

Theoretical literature

If you were to include empirical research only in your project, you would have lots of interesting findings, taken from systematic observations and experiments, but you would not be able to generalize or transfer these findings beyond your study. Undertaking a review of the theoretical literature enables you to consider the theories, ideas and concepts that might shed light on the results of your empirical literature review. You can then use these theories to explain your results and findings, and possibly generalize or transfer your findings to other contexts where this is appropriate. Without theories, you have lots of interesting findings but nothing to understand or interpret them with. When you include a review of the theoretical literature, you can incorporate your own findings with existing theories, ideas and concepts that may enable you to make some predictions and even develop the theories you have used. Theories are important as they provide a structure for your academic work, without which your ideas, even those gained from the empirical literature, are 'free floating' and cannot be easily applied to other contexts. In some literature reviews, you will be testing theories. When a theory is broken down into very small components, this might be referred to as a hypothesis:

- A *theory* is a well-established principle that explains some aspect of the natural world
- A *hypothesis* is a specific and testable prediction about what you expect to happen.

In other literature reviews, you will be generating theories. Theories provide a link between the different research you bring together in your review and possible explanations for the ideas created. Without supporting theories, even something quite simple (as in the example below), it is hard to argue that your ideas are generalizable or transferable to another situation.

Example
Hastings (2025) undertook a systematic review to understand what leads to organizational change within the healthcare environment. He provides three reasons for the approach to this review method: first, qualitative methods are generally used in organizational research; second, he used the Joanne Briggs Institute taxonomy for qualitative evidence synthesis; and third, he selected cases that included multiple transformations. He then reviewed the existing and dominant theories, including models and frameworks, and then compared these theories with the findings of the research that met the inclusion criteria for his review. This enabled him to compare the reality with the espoused theory.

So, it is important to be clear about what we mean by theory. The term theory is often used liberally in our everyday language. We might say 'in theory this should happen, but in practice ...', indicating a gap between the ideal and the real world. For example, we also often refer to the 'theory component' of a health or social care course, which generally refers to a body of knowledge that is used to underpin the taught practical content.

There is also a more specific understanding of the term theory which we use in research and academic traditions, in which the term theory refers to connecting patterns and concepts so that predictions and explanations can be made about how things work and what might happen (Wallace and Wray 2021). The term theory used in this way is a means of connecting concepts so that our understanding of the world increases and generalizations can be made. This understanding – or theory – might be developed via patterns observed through either actual empirical observations or 'armchair' theorizing (Wallace and Wray 2021), and may incorporate abstract and general thinking. Some theories will be well supported by empirical evidence and others will not be and may be refuted. Substantial theories are important in any academic piece of work as they demonstrate an academic depth and rigour to the study, and provide evidence that the researcher is able to apply the findings of the research to relevant contemporary theoretical concepts.

Theories are simplifications of the way the world works. Not all theories have names. They are not necessarily erudite constructions. The theory or hypothesis mentioned in the example concerning whether early detection of cancer saves lives cannot be attributed to any one individual, although many scientists have worked to develop this theory. Other theories are attributable to certain individuals – for example, Einstein's theory of relativity.

Theory refers to our general and abstract understanding about a topic rather than that merely provided by the empirical literature. While the empirical literature explores what actually happens in the real world in a specific context, the theoretical literature draws these observations together in an attempt to explain aspects of the social or physical world, in order to make predictions about what is likely to happen. Empirical studies may be guided implicitly or explicitly by theoretical constructs. Some empirical studies aim explicitly to test competing theories, but all use theories to interpret their findings. Theories are essential to the work of researchers as they provide an explanatory framework through which the results of empirical research can be interpreted and provide a way of generalizing or transferring the results.

Before you can explore possible theories that you may include in your literature review, you need to be clear about the exact terms and concepts you are referring to.

Defining the concepts used in your literature review

When you are doing a literature review, it is fundamental to your emerging study that you are familiar with the body of knowledge that underpins your topic and that you define the terms and concepts you are using in your review. These will usually be the terms and concepts that are stated in your literature review question but there might be other terms you need to explore and clarify. So, for example, if your literature review concerns the role played by spirituality in the psychodynamic approach to counselling (we have deliberately chosen this question as it is a complex example), you would need to define the concepts of spirituality and psychodynamic counselling, which in itself would be challenging.

Exploration of the concepts used will usually involve a comparison of the different ways in which they have been used in the existing literature. You might undertake a concept analysis or scoping study to do this. You might also undertake a focused mapping review and synthesis as outlined in Chapter 2. These options are considered by Mounce et al. (2024). Once you have reviewed the use of the concept, you need to commit to one understanding of the concept, even if the choice of definition you use feels somewhat arbitrary. You may consider that the concepts you use are clear and do not require further definition or clarification; however, it is essential to clarify their meaning and the conceptual underpinnings so that you can use them within your literature review.

Inclusion of theoretical literature in your literature review

During your post-graduate study, you are encouraged to identify theories and concepts that are relevant to your thesis as a whole. It is important to recognize what is a theory and what is not, referring back to the work of Wallace and Wray (2021) and to distinguish theories from the empirical findings.

Theories are likely to be explored initially in a background section of your project and returned to again once you have analysed your data in the discussion. This is the standard format for most literature reviews and empirical studies. However, if you are using qualitative methods such as grounded theory, your examination of theory will often be made once you have commenced the collection and analysis of your data rather than be identified at the beginning of the study. This is because when you undertake this type of exploratory study, you are generally seeking to generate theory rather than to test it, so it is unusual to commence the study with explicit reference to theory. This is in order not to lead the data analysis and to keep an open mind about the emerging results of the study. Instead, reference to relevant theory will emerge as the analysis progresses. However, you need to be aware of potential implicit theoretical concepts that you may hold as these may become a source of bias in your analysis.

- When your literature review is supportive and a prerequisite to a larger empirical study, relevant theories will be identified in the supporting literature review and often referred to in the analysis and interpretation of empirical data. There are some exceptions to this: for example, if you are undertaking a study as previously explained, perhaps a grounded theory study, and are developing your own theory, in which case you would avoid seeking out established theory prior to undertaking your own study.

- When your literature review is a standalone literature review, relevant theories will often be explored in the introduction and then referred to in the analysis and interpretations of the literature reviewed.

Searching for relevant theories

Searching for relevant theories can be a complex process, which we will discuss in detail in Chapter 4. Indeed, Booth and Carroll (2015) noted that the process of searching for theories was not articulated in many works identified for the purposes of their study. That is, while there is agreement that research studies should refer to relevant theories, these are not so easily articulated. There are several reasons why searching for theories is problematic. Some theories are searchable by name, while others are more elusive. Theories will often be identified through wide reading and knowledge of the key texts and researchers in your area. The theoretical literature available can be vast and may vary in quality and scope.

Understanding competing theories

It is likely that you will find one or more competing theories about the topic you are studying. Theories come into and go out of fashion and are adapted as we gain understanding through empirical observation.

> In physics, there are mainline theories that many people might assume are firmly established. Yet even these are often refined. The ongoing search for a 'Grand Unified Theory', which could explain everything, would probably change any theories we currently have. Therefore, no theory is set in stone.

Some theories will be robust and supported by strong empirical evidence, while others will be less well supported and may be rejected. Further empirical evidence may enhance or decrease support for a theory and theoretical development. Often empirical research will test out, refine and develop new theories. Some theories can be no more than a hunch or an idea. For example, one very early theory that 'the world is flat' dominated the thinking of many early civilizations until advancements in science and travel led to its revision.

Theories develop as our knowledge develops. In health and social care, this is usually as a result of the advancement of knowledge through empirical studies. So, for example, there is the very well-known and established theory that smoking causes lung cancer. Most people would now accept that the possibility that this theory will be rejected is extremely unlikely. However, it was the increase in empirical studies exploring the link between tobacco and lung cancer in the 1950s and 1960s that supported the development of this causal theory.

It is common to find theories that compete with each other. Take, for example, the theory of behaviour change, as described by Prochaska et al. (1994). This theory states that people work through a series of predefined stages during the process of behaviour change, for example in smoking cessation (Prochaska et al. 1994), and was popular at the start of the twenty-first century. In contrast, West argued that the empirical evidence did not support the behaviour change theory. He developed the competing theory that many people do not work through a series of stages in order to change a behaviour but instead can make an overnight decision to break a habit (West 2006).

From the examples given above, you can see that incorporating theories into your review can be a complex process. Relevant theories might be hard to find and not easy to search for. They may not be as easily identified as other types of literature, as we shall explore in Chapter 4. You might perceive that you have identified them by chance through background reading, and some theoretical positions might only be implicitly stated in empirical papers. You are likely to encounter many possible theories, including some which compete with one another.

Example of how researchers have used theories to support the design of a quantitative study

Frie et al. (2020) undertook a PhD study in which they explored the use of self-monitoring of weight as a weight management strategy. People who want to lose weight are often advised to closely monitor their weight. Self-monitoring of weight is an essential component of this and is associated with theories of self-regulation. Frie et al. were interested if further self-regulation activities could enhance weight loss. They used theories of self-regulation to help design their study. Applying these theories, they devised an RCT in which they compared standard self-monitoring of weight at home with an enhanced home weigh-in, which included different tasks that link to the different steps of the self-regulation process, including: (1) contextualizing the weight measurement, (2) reflecting on behaviour and (3) planning weight loss actions, while incorporating the theories of self-regulation and how these might be effectively applied to weight loss strategies.

The following is an extract from Frie et al. (2020: 17):

> *The effectiveness of self-monitoring is hypothesised to be based on a self-regulation process, whereby monitoring oneself allows for (1) the comparison of the current status to a previously set goal, thus providing (2) the opportunity to reflect on the effectiveness of previous behaviour, and enabling (3) the formulation of an action plan to reach the goal, which is followed by (4) the performance of the planned action (Boutelle, 2006; Kanfer & Karoly, 1972; LaRose et al., 2009).*

Example of how researchers have investigated behavioural theories in a review

Darukaradhya and Krishnamurthy (2025) were interested in examining the efficacy of behavioural theories for promoting health communication and behaviour change in non-communicable diseases. These types of diseases account for over 41 million deaths annually worldwide and for almost three-quarters of all morbidities. Thus, they are a major public health challenge and account for much of the care provided by health and social care workers. In the absence of effective treatments, behaviour change is an important strategy for prevention and lifestyle modification to reduce their impact. Psychologists and social scientists have developed a number of different theories to account for behaviour change and guide intervention development. Darukaradhya and Krishnamurthy (2025) reviewed the literature to examine four major groups of theory-driven behaviour change interventions, including those targeting intrapersonal factors, interpersonal factors, community factors and integrated models (combining all three factors). They identified 35 papers, with 27 studies demonstrating statistically significant benefits. Most studies used interpersonal or integrated models, and the authors concluded that these theories provided the best evidence of efficacy.

The above two examples illustrate how you might incorporate theories in your project and use them to develop your ideas and arguments. The theories you identify will require a judgement about their relevance. It is not always possible to get a complete or exhaustive picture of all the potentially relevant theories that are associated with your research question or topic. Any topic could be informed by many different theories. You will usually engage with the theories that are relevant to your academic discipline. So, for example, if your project is situated within psychology, you are likely to refer to psychological theories rather than sociological theories even though some sociological theories might have clear relevance to your work.

If you are doing a PhD or doctoral-level study, your engagement with theories and concepts will be more extensive than if you were studying at master's level. However, at master's level you would usually be expected to identify relevant theories that provide an explanatory framework for your project in a section of your literature review and to refer back to them in the discussion section of your dissertation. It is useful to explore some of the relevant theories so that you have an anchor upon which to develop your ideas as your study progresses. It is also important that you can discuss and critique the theoretical ideas you encounter. You need to be able to recognize which theories are relevant to your literature review and distinguish them from more general background information. It is also important that you can identify the extent to which the theories are supported by empirical literature and how relevant they are to your literature review.

Methodological literature

Methodological literature refers to those papers (or aspects of papers) that investigate or describe research methods and practices. You might come across a paper that focuses solely on the discussion of methods used in a study reported elsewhere, or you might find a detailed discussion of methods used within a study which also reports the findings of the empirical research. Methodological literature is important in many ways when you are considering the literature that informs your ongoing project.

You will get a feel for the type of research that has been carried out in your area and this may enable you to do a more focused or refined search for further research of this kind. This might help with your search strategy, which we will discuss in Chapter 4. Focusing on the methodological aspects of a study will help you to understand and critically evaluate the research methods used by other researchers whose work you are using and critiquing in your review. We will discuss this further in Chapters 5 and 6.

Most importantly, however, the examination of the methods used in empirical studies might also help you to select and justify what methods to use for your own study. Reviewing the methods of published research can help you establish and decide upon your own method for your research – be it a standalone literature review or a larger empirical study if appropriate.

- When the literature review is supportive and a prerequisite to a larger empirical study, methodological literature may be used to identify suitable methods for the empirical study. You can critique the methods used in the papers you identify for your review in order to help you identify appropriate research methods.
- When the literature review is a standalone review, the methodological literature can be used to justify the approach you take to your literature review method. You may also use the methodological literature to comment on the research approaches used in the literature you include in your review.

Example

When we were writing this book, much scrutiny was given to the methods used in undertaking various types of literature reviews. We have scrutinized the methods sections of research papers and contacted researchers to get a better insight as to why they used the methods they reported. This focus on the way different researchers used the literature review methods enabled us to consider the consistency with which different approaches were used and to build a picture of the common features occurring in most literature reviews. You can use the methodological literature to justify overarching approaches, such as a literature review method, or individual methods within a research design, such as approaches to interviewing.

Inclusion of methodological literature in your literature review

If your literature review is a prerequisite to a larger empirical study, you are likely to refer to the existing literature that explores research methods in order to develop the appropriate research methods for your own study. Depending on your study, you might devote an entire section of your literature review to the discussion of relevant methodological issues. This literature will not necessarily be a separate set of papers.

By the time you have searched for literature in your research area (which we discuss in Chapter 4), you are likely to have a body of empirical material documenting the studies that are relevant to your research. When you read empirical studies related to your own research area, it is useful to consider more than just the findings of the empirical results of those studies. In addition to using these studies to inform your knowledge about previous work that has been undertaken, you can use this literature to identify *how* previous research has been undertaken and how researchers evaluated their use of these methods. You can examine the details of the methods and evaluations of these methods by researchers to help you refine the method for your own study. You can then refer to and/or review these methods and take notice of their limitations to help you develop your own methods for your empirical study.

To start with, you are likely to examine the research methods used in the empirical research you have already identified as relevant to your research area, but it might also be useful to examine research methods of studies that are not directly related to your review or subsequent empirical study but where the methods might be transferable. Depending on how you use the empirical literature, some additional searches related to methods may be required, especially if you draw on studies that you are not using in your empirical literature review.

Using literature about methods to shape the design of your study

Papers identified in a literature review can help you shape and design the research methods you use in your study. You are most likely to do this if your literature review is 'supportive' to a larger study in which you are developing methods to use in your empirical study. However, if your literature review is a standalone review, you will need to justify the approach you have chosen to undertake your own literature review.

> Some researchers might put the discussion of methodological aspects of the research in the methodology section of their thesis. Others might put it in the literature review section. It is up to individual researchers to decide where this section best fits into their work but the focus needs to be clear that the review of empirical literature is undertaken in order to assess the methods used in order to inform the methods used in your own study.

We will use some examples from the literature review section of three reviews to illustrate how the methodological literature has been used to inform the development of research methods for a larger empirical study.

Example of how researchers used literature about methods to justify the use of interviews in their study

Research papers that describe their methods in detail, or methodological literature that focuses solely on methods, can be used to identify methods which have been used previously in research similar to that in your own study. These methods can then be considered to see if they are suitable and relevant methods that might help you address your research question.

For example, Alzyood et al. (2020) undertook a research study to explore the potential role of patients in promoting handwashing – patient prompting of handwashing can be regarded as part of the wider involvement of patients in a safety initiative. However, if patients are to be encouraged to prompt handwashing, it is important to understand if this is a behaviour that is acceptable to both patients and nurses alike. A review of the literature identified that while many surveys had been conducted on both nurses' and patients' perceptions of patient prompting of handwashing, very few had explored this in depth (Alzyood et al. 2018). While the surveys went some way in describing the perceptions and to some extent the experiences of patients and nurses regarding patient prompting of handwashing, there was no depth to the findings, as might be expected from such an approach. Surveys did not give an in-depth understanding of what happens when patients prompt nurses to wash their hands. The benefits of using surveys included that they were relatively easy to administer and they did not expose either the nurse or patient to difficult conversations. The disadvantage of using surveys was that the depth of understanding of experience remained largely unexplored.

This example illustrates how the empirical literature enabled the researchers to identify and justify appropriate research methods for a proposed study. Interviews with nurses and patients were identified as the most appropriate way to collect more in-depth data around the issue of patient prompting of handwashing. Use of the methodological literature in this example not only helped the researchers to identify a gap in the research regarding a lack of in-depth understanding of experience but also helped them to identify appropriate ways in which this situation might be discussed in interviews.

Example of how researchers used papers that discuss methods to identify a method of measurement in their study

Methodological literature can be used to identify methods of undertaking an intervention to be used in a study and how a certain type of measurement can be obtained.

For example, a research study was undertaken to determine the optimum management in clinical practice of the build-up of ascites in patients with a malignancy (Preston 2004). The management of ascites refers to clinicians' attempts to deal with the large volume of fluid that can build up in the peritoneal (abdominal) cavity. This research was undertaken to explore how this process could be managed most effectively and acceptably for the patient. A vital part of the research was the measurement of pressure in the intra-peritoneal cavity. It was important to determine the best way of measuring this. A literature review had been conducted to identify papers that recorded ways of measuring intra-abdominal pressure. The review identified that the main method applied had been to use an approximation for abdominal pressure rather than to measure it directly. In order to do this, the patient is given pressure-sensitive telemetry pills to swallow and an approximation of abdominal pressure is made from the stomach. However, this process is not an exact simulation for abdominal ascites as the stomach is a muscular structure that undergoes constriction itself, which can result in a change of pressure. The researcher felt that this approach was suboptimal and that direct measurement, in which the peritoneal cavity is accessed through a drainage tube, was preferable. This should have been possible using a narrow pressure transducer, which could be fed down the tube used to drain the ascites. However, what was unknown was the pressure range that the pressure transducer needed to be sensitive to. A subsequent review of the literature was undertaken in order to estimate upper and lower pressure ranges from indirect measurements. As a result, an upper limit was set and a transducer purchased that was sensitive enough to show changes in pressure slightly beyond this upper limit (Preston 2004).

This example illustrates how the methodological literature can be used for guidance about how to obtain measurements that are required in a research project. It also illustrates how the knowledge and understanding obtained by previous researchers can enhance the method of future studies.

Example of how researchers used papers that discuss methods to develop strategies for recruitment in their study

Methodological literature can be used to determine the most effective ways to recruit participants into a study.

For example, McCallum et al. (2019) undertook a review of the literature on the recruitment into research of individuals who had recently been bereaved, a group of people who are often perceived to be vulnerable and therefore 'hard to reach'. The authors identified a selection of papers in which people who had experienced a bereavement had been invited to take part in a study. The researchers scrutinized the methods by which they had been invited and looked for evidence of their acceptability to the invitees based on the assumption that, had any methods been considered inappropriate this would have been documented in the paper. McCallum et al. identified a range of strategies used to invite the recently bereaved into studies and used these to argue for their chosen approach when seeking ethical approval.

The above examples illustrate how the scrutiny of the methods used by other researchers can help inform the choice you make about methodological decisions in your own project. These should be written up when you discuss the research methods you selected in your study. You can discuss the ways in which you referred to the work of others, research methods you found helpful and those you chose not to use.

In summary

It is important to remember to frame your project within the existing empirical, theoretical and methodological work that has been undertaken in your topic area. Your study will not achieve its full potential until you can demonstrate how your review relates to other work in the area. The phrase 'standing on the shoulders of giants' is applicable here.

At all levels of study, your engagement with the empirical research literature is likely to be the main emphasis of your literature review. Drawing on the existing empirical work that informs the area is a central feature of undertaking a literature review. However, it is also important to draw on the work of others who have engaged with theories, ideas and concepts that are related to your area and the methods that others have used in their studies, in order to help you develop your methods for your review and subsequent empirical study where applicable.

If you are doing a PhD or doctoral-level study, your review of the empirical, theoretical and methodological literature will be more extensive than for students studying at master's level, and you need to make a judgement, in collaboration with your supervisor, about the level of engagement that is appropriate for your study.

In the next chapter, we will discuss how you can search for empirical, theoretical and methodological literature.

Key points

- In all post-graduate study, it is important to set your work within the context of others
- This includes review of theories and methods in addition to the empirical literature
- Empirical literature will enable you to discuss the existing research
- Theoretical literature will enable you to explore theories, concepts and ideas
- Methodological literature will enable you to explore possible research methods to inform your study.

4

How do I search for relevant literature?

In this chapter, we will discuss:

- *Why a comprehensive search strategy is important*
- *When you might use different approaches to searching*
- *How to search electronic databases*
- *How to employ additional search strategies.*

In this chapter, we will explore how you search for the different types of literature that you may include in your review. We will discuss this with reference to searching for empirical, theoretical and methodological literature.

When you identify your question for your literature review, you will determine inclusion and exclusion criteria that will enable you to focus your search. Your search will be directed by your review question and the criteria for inclusion you set.

How comprehensive does my search need to be?

At first, you might think that you need to identify every possible piece of literature that is relevant to your review. In reality, you need to think carefully about the scope of your review so that you move quickly from the selection of very general to the specific research and other evidence that is relevant to your project. You are unlikely to have the time or the word count in your thesis to cover more general issues related to your project and, if you do, this is likely to be at the expense of the more detailed examination of research and other evidence that is directly relevant to your study. Focusing in on the literature that is specifically relevant to your project requires a judgement as you clearly need to set the context of your study. It is important to remember that you are likely to be limited by a thesis word count and you cannot afford to 'waste' words on generic matters relating to your topic; you need to focus on the specific area you are researching as soon as possible. You are likely to include more general background information in an introduction. We will discuss this further in Chapter 8 when we consider the art and science of writing up a literature review.

Comprehensive searching

Once you have established the specific focus of your review, your review question and inclusion and exclusion criteria, your search for relevant literature that meets these criteria will usually – but not always – be comprehensive.

Example
McCallum et al. (2019) undertook a PhD study in which they explored the experiences of family members of people who died in the emergency department. This literature review was therefore a prerequisite to a larger empirical study. The main focus of their literature review was empirical research that had been undertaken by previous researchers who had investigated the experiences of family members who had been in this situation. For this section of the literature review, the researchers conducted a comprehensive search as it was essential that they identified all the studies that had previously been undertaken which related directly to their study focus – that is, which met their inclusion criteria. Any omissions might have led to a gap in the review and hence incomplete conclusions could have been drawn that could have affected the subsequent empirical study.

This type of comprehensive approach to literature searching is sometimes referred to as an 'exhaustive' approach. In this type of search, it is important that you identify all relevant research or other evidence so that your review is comprehensive and does not omit significant work in the area, as discussed in Chapter 1. This is the approach advocated by the Cochrane Collaboration, and it requires that researchers obtain all available empirical evidence that addresses the literature review (or systematic review) question. Specific advice in the Cochrane Handbook is that literature reviewers should:

> *attempt to collate all empirical evidence that fits pre-existing eligibility criteria in order to answer a specific research question … systematic methods that are selected with a view to minimising bias, thus providing more reliable findings from which conclusions can be drawn and decisions made.*
>
> (Higgins et al. 2024)

There is general agreement as to what is understood by a comprehensive search (Cooper et al. 2018). There is some debate as to whether such a search is needed for all reviews. Given that it arose from the methods for doing a Cochrane systematic review with meta-analysis, where evidence for effectiveness is sought, the need for a comprehensive search in other reviews where in-depth understanding is sought might be questioned. Indeed, the Centre for Reviews and Dissemination (2008), Tong et al. (2012) and Hannes and Macaitis (2012) discuss the lack of consensus for undertaking a comprehensive search for all review types. Tong et al. (2012) refer to the concept of 'theoretical saturation', where a concept is comprehensively reviewed even if not all the papers have been reviewed. Yet not undertaking a comprehensive search risks omitting relevant literature and 'cherry picking' papers for review. We suggest that at postgraduate level, you endeavour to undertake an exhaustive or comprehensive search for the research and other evidence that addresses your empirical review question and that meets your inclusion and exclusion criteria, unless your supervisory team advises otherwise. Where an exhaustive search is not feasible, you should undertake as comprehensive a search as is reasonable within the limitations of your resources for your project. This is because, in your literature review, you are seeking to find every relevant piece of literature in order to avoid 'cherry picking' evidence and omitting vital research, which could potentially bias or affect the review. Your aim is to identify all the available literature that might contribute to answering your literature review question.

This involves explicit planning of the exact focus of the review, key terms and synonyms, and identifying appropriate databases. The literature search usually extends beyond a database search and includes other strategies for identifying appropriate literature – such as reference list searching, citation tracking and contacting key researchers – so that no stone is left unturned in the search for literature, including any that is unpublished. We discuss additional strategies for identifying literature later in this chapter. At the time of writing, whilst it might provide some relevant references, artificial intelligence (AI) cannot replicate a comprehensive search.

Although your search should usually be comprehensive, it is important to note that not everything will be incorporated into the results of your review. Much of the research and other evidence you identify will be filtered out by inclusion and exclusion criteria so that anything you do include is directly relevant to your review. These inclusion and exclusion criteria will include considerations of relevance, quality or appropriateness of research method, and will be justified with a clear rationale, which we will discuss later in the chapter. Sometimes the inclusion criteria will specify particular research methods for inclusion in the study. For example, in Cochrane Collaboration reviews of effectiveness, the review protocols may specify that only RCTs are included as these are considered to be the best evidence for this type of review. In addition, other quality criteria are sometimes applied so that only the very 'best available' evidence is included. For example, you may decide to include only interview-based studies rather than questionnaires if your review is of a particularly sensitive topic and you do not feel that data from questionnaires will have sufficient depth to be relevant. This will depend on the review in question, and a judgement will need to be made by the reviewers as to the inclusion and exclusion criteria set.

Selective or purposive searching

The alternative to a fully comprehensive search for literature is a selective or purposive search. This might also be referred to as theoretical sampling. In this approach, researchers do not seek to identify all literature but search for a selection of literature that meets the needs of the review. Whilst the concept of selective or purposive sampling is securely established within qualitative research, it is treated with caution when discussed in the context of literature reviews. This is because the purpose of a review is almost always to review the entire body of evidence rather than a sample of it, which may not be representative of the whole. However, this approach may be adopted in certain large-scale qualitative and mixed-methods reviews where the literature review is a standalone study and where the aim of the review is interpretive rather than aggregative or summative. In this case, reviewers often aim to develop concepts or to capture the main themes arising in a body of literature, and cease searching when new literature does not add to conceptual clarity, understanding or knowledge development. This is an approach advocated by Noblit and Hare (1988), Dixon-Woods et al. (2005) and Thomas and Harden (2008).

For example, in what was the first Cochrane qualitative systematic review, in which Glenton et al. (2013) reported the barriers and facilitators to the implementation by lay health workers of improving access to maternal and child health, the authors used a purposive or selective approach to the literature included in their study. They extracted data from the results of the included qualitative studies. Glenton et al. (2013) noted that it is not always practical to analyse large amounts of qualitative research in the depth required to avoid a simplistic overview, and they described how too many studies can threaten the quality of data analysis. In recent years, however, even researchers who have used a method for undertaking a literature review (e.g. meta-ethnography) where purposive sampling is suggested have erred on the side of caution and undertaken a comprehensive search. The meta-ethnographic review by Leufstadius et al. (2024) is an example of this.

For the purposes of this book, we argue that purposive or selective searching should not be undertaken by anyone doing a literature review without a strong rationale. It is generally restricted to those undertaking a large-scale standalone qualitative or mixed-methods review who have made a judgement that a comprehensive search is not appropriate in their particular case. This is a judgement that needs to be defended when writing up the method undertaken for the review or in the oral examination.

Selective or purposive searching may be relevant when you are searching for additional methodological and theoretical literature to supplement the literature you have already identified in your comprehensive search. Searching for theories can be a complex process, even if you commence your project with a clear idea of the theories you will be referring to in your work. You are unlikely to be required to identify all the possible theories that might relate to your project – unless the specific demands of your project require this. You are expected to identify relevant theories that can help you to explain the data that you analyse in your review. The process of searching for theories is likely to be iterative as different theories may be explored and reviewed for the contribution they make to the understanding of the research question. Similarly, the search for methodological literature does not need to be comprehensive, as researchers are looking for examples and justification for the approaches taken to research design. The aim of referring to the supporting methodological literature is to provide examples and justification for the research methods you have chosen rather than to provide a comprehensive discussion of all possible appropriate methods.

Additional searches

Whichever strategy you employ in your search for research and other evidence, you will likely need to undertake supplementary searches for theoretical and methodological literature as the needs of your project demand (Table 4.1). These searches will be additional to the comprehensive search you will have undertaken. These searches might also 'snowball' from the existing literature identified from your comprehensive search (Greenhalgh and Peacock 2005), such as from reading lists of identified studies.

Table 4.1 How inclusive does my literature search need to be?

<table>
<tr><th></th><th>Research and other evidence that meet your inclusion and exclusion criteria</th><th>Supporting theoretical literature</th><th>Supporting methodological literature</th></tr>
<tr><td>Your main project is an empirical study. The literature review is a supportive literature review</td><td rowspan="2">Usually, you should aim to include all empirical research and other evidence that meets your inclusion and exclusion criteria for your literature review question</td><td rowspan="2">You should aim to Discuss the main theories, concepts and ideas that relate to your research question in some detail</td><td>You should aim to refer to the methods used by other researchers who have researched similar areas or participant groups to justify the methods you adopt for your study</td></tr>
<tr><td>Your main project is a literature review from which you hope to answer a research question. We will refer to this as a standalone literature review</td><td>If your main project is a literature review, you are likely to include a rationale for the approach to the literature review you have chosen (e.g. systematic review, meta-ethnographic review)</td></tr>
</table>

The search strategy

For some literature reviews, including Cochrane systematic reviews with meta-analysis, the search strategy is completely pre-defined. The search strategy will have been tested in advance and, once established, it is the one that is used and often formally updated every three to five years. In other reviews, the search strategy will evolve as the project proceeds in a more iterative manner. Chapman et al. (2009) noted that searching is also often conducted in several phases and is not a linear process. The search strategy may not be pre-defined in specific detail but emerges as the literature is identified, and investigation of one area of literature might lead to exploration of further literature. Finfgeld-Connett and Johnson (2013) argued that searching is not a linear or 'one-off' process and cannot be determined accurately at the start of a project. In fact, some proponents of the approach argue that prior planning and the pre-definition of all terms may preclude creativity and thinking about the concepts, thus possibly inhibiting their development. Therefore, in some projects, you may return to the databases for additional searches when the need becomes apparent as you progress with your project. Interestingly, despite the emergence of a wide range of approaches to doing a literature review, most of these approaches do not outline a specific approach to the process of searching (Sutton et al. 2019).

Developing a search strategy

Whichever approach you choose, searching is often harder than it looks. What seems to be an intuitive process can be far more complex. Take the example of van Hoorn et al. (2016), who wished to explore optimum search strategies for studies on patient preferences regarding treatment outcomes; the researchers commenced their study by addressing how to search for appropriate literature. Therefore, once you have established the purpose of your literature review and your approach to searching, you need to develop a search strategy that is carefully considered and appropriate to the requirements of your project, and which will enable you to identify and locate the most relevant range of published and unpublished material (where relevant) to answer your research question.

Specialist librarian input

You are strongly advised to consult an academic librarian to assist you with developing your search strategy. Your university, hospital library or professional body may be able to assist you in seeking advice from a specialist librarian. However, remember that you will be required to defend your approach to searching either in your written thesis or in an oral examination, and you should not delegate the task of searching to a third party. It is your project and you need to maintain control of the process. When you consult a specialist librarian, ensure that they are aware that you are searching for a literature review and that you are looking for everything that addresses your question in the first instance (unless you have made a conscious decision not to do this, as discussed earlier in the chapter), rather than a more refined and manageable list of possible references. It is important to remember that there is a difference between writing an essay, where you are interested in relevant references on your topic, and writing a literature review, where you are interested in all the references on your topic. Specialist librarians are trained to guide researchers and professionals towards both of these options and you therefore need to be specific about the needs of your individual project when discussing your search strategy. If resources permit, academic librarians can peer review your search strategy (McGowan et al. 2016; Duffy and Lefebvre 2023); developing your search strategy can be a complex task and one that can benefit from discussion with others to check for logic and inclusivity in search terms. If you are unable to liaise with your academic librarian, then working alongside a colleague to check your search strategy is another good approach.

Defining key terms

When searching for research and other evidence related to your literature review question, the first step is to identify the key terms under which research and other evidence may be identified in an electronic database and with which you would recognize the potentially relevant titles and abstracts stored in that database. The reason behind identifying key terms is that when journal articles are entered onto a database, their key terms are stored there. When the same key terms are entered into that database, the relevant articles will be retrieved.

Key terms are the important words or ideas in your literature review question that should be included in an article you are looking for, in order for it to be relevant to you. Key terms are either identified by you as the researcher or they can be identified from a pre-prepared list – for example, as subject headings, MeSH (medical subject heading) terms or thesaurus terms – which you will find listed within the database. We will discuss both of these options later in the chapter. Each database works slightly differently and it is important to become familiar with the database you are searching so that you can search using your own key terms or those pre-identified in the subject headings (or equivalent).

Key terms and synonyms

In addition to key terms, it is also necessary to identify as many synonyms – words that mean the same thing as the key term – as possible. This maximizes your chances of finding research and other evidence that may use different terminology but which nonetheless is relevant to your literature review. It is important that your key terms and synonyms should be as comprehensive as possible, while not deviating too much from the original term for which you are searching. Key terms can be identified by a simple 'brainstorm' of relevant phrases that might be used in connection with your topic, including words no longer currently in use. Ideas for key terms can also be identified from papers that you have already consulted, or can be obtained using simple Google searches that link you to other general information on your review question. Artificial intelligence (AI) can be used to help you identify synonyms but use your judgement as to whether these are appropriate or not. You may be able to use search terms used in previous studies; for example, Cochrane systematic reviews with meta-analysis have very well-developed search terms, with strings of terms for specific searches. Care and consideration is needed when identifying key terms. For example, the key term 'qualitative' will not necessarily access all qualitative research as many databases will not have always recognized this term (Noyes and Popay 2007). Furthermore, the term 'qualitative' is broad and is likely to identify papers unrelated to qualitative research.

Tools to assist the development of key terms

In addition to the strategies mentioned above for the identification of key terms, various tools or acronyms have been developed to facilitate the identification of an appropriate range of key terms and synonyms. One of the most well-known is the PICO (Population, Intervention, Comparison, Outcome) tool, widely used by researchers to define their research question and hence their search strategy. PICO has been adopted by the Cochrane Collaboration (Cooke et al. 2012) as a guide to both the formulation of the research question and the identification of key terms and synonyms. The origins of the PICO tool can be traced back to the early discussion about evidence-based practice (Richardson 1998) and the importance of asking a clearly focused question with clearly defined elements. Richardson (1998) identified that good clinical questions generally contain three or four well-defined elements and these have become the basis of the PICO acronym. Using this acronym as a trigger, researchers are encouraged to identify a key term and relevant alternative terms or synonyms for the population, intervention, comparison and outcomes appropriate to their literature review question. The version of PICO described above has its origins in the quantitative domain, with reference to interventions and comparisons. Alternative tools and acronyms have been developed that are considered to be more appropriate for literature review questions that are more qualitative in nature. Fineout-Overholt and Johnston (2005) discuss the adaptation of the PICO tool for qualitative research questions: Population, Issue, Context, Outcome. In this version, some of the 'quantitative' terms used in the original PICO version have been replaced with 'qualitative' terms: namely, intervention is replaced by issue and comparison is replaced by context.

Another tool or acronym is SPICE: Setting, Population, Intervention, Comparison, Evaluation. With this tool, Cooke et al. (2012) recognized the evaluative nature of qualitative research, with the addition of evaluation; however, the quantitative origins of the tool are still evident as the focus is on intervention and comparison. Another more qualitative tool is SPIDER: Sample, Phenomena of Interest, Design, Evaluation, Research type. In this tool, population is replaced by sample (Cooke et al. 2012) (see Table 4.2).

Which tool or acronym should I use?

The purpose of these acronyms is to enhance the identification of key terms and synonyms that will lead you to the most relevant references for your literature review. The aim of any tool is to trigger the identification of key terms and synonyms that might otherwise not be identified. Thus, use of the tool should trigger the most comprehensive search for literature.

Each of the different tools focuses on different elements of the research question and hence will place a different emphasis on the subsequent search strategy. In order to find out how effective these tools or acronyms are at triggering researchers to identify the most appropriate key terms and synonyms, a formal evaluation of each would be required. When you decide to use one of these tools, it is useful to consider the evaluations that have already been carried out. It is beyond the scope of this book to review the literature for tools and acronyms and their evaluations; however, two such evaluations of these tools have been identified.

Table 4.2 Different tools for identifying key terms

PICOT – quantitative (Higgins et al. 2024) • **P**opulation • **I**ntervention • **C**omparison • **O**utcome • **T**ime (not always included)
PICOT – qualitative (Fineout-Overholt and Johnston 2005) • **P**opulation • **I**ssue • **C**ontext • **O**utcome • **T**ime (not always included)
SPICE (Cooke et al. 2012) • **S**etting • **P**opulation • **I**ntervention • **C**ontrol • **E**valuation
SPIDER (Cooke et al. 2012) • **S**ample • **P**henomena of Interest • **D**esign • **E**valuation • **R**esearch
PEO (developed from PICOT) • **P**opulation • **E**xposure • **O**utcome

Cooke et al. (2012) and Methley et al. (2014) reviewed the effectiveness of the extent to which PICO, SPICE and SPIDER are both specific and sensitive in identifying appropriate literature for a qualitative evidence synthesis. Cooke et al. (2012) found that PICO provided the most comprehensive range of results when the key terms and synonyms were combined in a database search. The use of SPIDER led to a specific but less comprehensive range of results, which could be useful for purposive or selective searching but less useful when exhaustive or comprehensive searching is required. Methley et al. (2014) compared PICO, SPICE and SPIDER and also concluded that PICO provided the most comprehensive set of results, while SPICE and SPIDER led to a selection of literature. Evaluation of these tools is ongoing. It is unlikely that there will be one tool that is best for all literature reviews, and certainly no tool that will guarantee that you will identify all the literature that is relevant to your review question. You are advised to choose the tool whose terms seem the 'best fit' to your study. The most important thing is that the tool enables you to identify a comprehensive range of key terms and synonyms (Tables 4.3 and 4.4). You might find that a combination of the concepts identified in the tools will facilitate this.

Table 4.3 Identifying key terms and synonyms using PICO (quantitative version)

Literature review question: 'Is morphine effective in reducing pain in end-of-life care?'

	Population	**Intervention**	**Comparison**	**Outcome**
PICO term	Palliative care	Morphine	Non-opioids	Reduced pain on pain scale
Alternative terms (synonyms)	Terminal End of life Supportive	Oramorph Narcotic Heroin	Paracetamol NSAID Ibuprofen	Patient comfort Assessment Pain rating scale

Table 4.4 Identifying key terms and synonyms using PICO (qualitative version)

Literature review question: 'Are relatives consulted about pain relief in end-of-life care settings?'

	Population	**Issue**	**Context**	**Outcome**
PICO term	Relatives	Pain relief	End-of-life care settings	Experience
Alternative terms (synonyms)	Family Caregivers Carers Next of kin	Analgesia Narcotics	Hospice Palliative care unit Terminal care	Feelings Thoughts Perceptions

Electronic database searching

Once you have identified your key terms and synonyms, the next step is to plan your electronic database search. The main approach for all searches is likely to be via electronic databases. There are a vast number of databases that will give you access to a range of different journals. A thorough investigation of available databases will enable you to access the most appropriate for your review. Some databases are specific to the academic discipline you work within. Some are also freely available without a subscription. At the time of writing, it is not possible for AI to replace the process of searching. Artificial intelligence does not have access to the databases and the nuances of searching require judgement not currently available with AI tools.

Most academic and hospital libraries will provide a list of databases they subscribe to, together with a description of their content. The names of databases are usually accompanied by a description of each so that you can assess whether it is likely to be relevant to your work. As the availability of databases and their content change on a frequent basis, you are advised to go directly to your academic or hospital library to identify which databases might be appropriate for your search.

Commonly used databases include:

- MEDLINE and PUBMED: extensive medical, nursing and allied health database
- CINAHL: nursing and allied healthcare with a North American and European focus
- EThOS: PhD thesis database
- ZETOC, Open Grey, NHS evidence: databases of grey literature
- PsycINFO: psychology, psychiatry and child development
- Web of Science: includes Science Citation Index and Social Science Citation Index.

Try to identify as many databases as you can that contain material relevant to your literature review. This will maximize your chances of identifying appropriate and relevant research and other evidence for your review. We strongly recommend that you avoid using Google or Google Scholar because these search engines have access to a vast amount of literature that will not be relevant to you and have limited access to academic resources, and hence you are likely to be inundated with many irrelevant hits. Limiting your search to Google and Google Scholar will restrict your attempt to identify all the relevant research and other evidence on your topic. However, Google Scholar can be useful for initial searches in order to assist you with the identification of key terms as well as useful for citation searching, which we discuss later. Google or Google Scholar can also be useful in retrieving full-text copies of papers that you have located through more comprehensive database searches but for which the full copy of the paper is not otherwise accessible. Note that it is often possible to request a full copy from another library, but there is likely to be a cost for this service. You can also use Research Gate to identify papers or you can contact the authors directly.

Basics of database searching

It is important that you develop good database searching skills. This is a complex process and needs practice to refine and time to consider how you might formulate the best search strategies. The aim of database searching is that you identify references to research and other evidence that may be relevant to your literature review question. These references are often referred to as 'hits'.

Ideally, your searching on electronic databases will be sensitive enough that you do not identify a large number of irrelevant references and specific enough that you identify papers (hits) that are appropriate for your review.

- If your search is too specific and too sensitive, you will sense that you have only seen the 'tip of the iceberg' and that there are many unlocated hits that might be relevant for your review.
- If your search is not sufficiently specific or sensitive, you will be inundated with references (hits) that are not relevant for your review.

Clearly, you should aim for a middle road that enables you to identify appropriate references from a wider list that is not too extensive. Achieving this requires a certain level of skill.

There are two approaches to database searching. The first is to use the key terms and synonyms you have identified in a 'free-text' search, using the search boxes in the databases. This type of search enables you to use all the key terms you have identified and to be creative about adding new terms to the search as and when they appear, if this fits with your search protocol. You can also choose to search for your key term in the title, abstract or full text, giving you flexibility over the search process. For example, if you are searching for a term that is likely to be given only a brief mention in a paper, then a full-text search will pick this up, whereas a search in which the key term was limited to the title or abstract would not. Equally, limiting your search to those papers in which the key term appears in the title or abstract is a useful strategy if you are fairly confident that the key term and the focus of the paper are likely to be similar.

> Hooley et al. (2024) illustrate the balance required between garnering too many and not enough hits. They describe how, in their study, including key terms such as 'communication' and 'advanced care planning' led to far too many hits and a decision had to be made about more specific search terms.

The second approach to database searching is to undertake a 'controlled search' using subject headings that have been pre-identified on the database you are using. These are often referred to as MeSH or subject headings, but other terms might be used, depending on which database you are using. A controlled search uses subject headings as key terms that have been identified by the people compiling the database in order to facilitate the indexing of papers. If you use a controlled search, you will identify papers with key terms that correspond to the pre-identified term. Searching in this way is likely to enable you to locate specific literature but also lead you to fewer papers, as indexing is limited by the perspective of the professional indexers who are entering papers into the database. The search will also be limited to published papers where the key term is already identified as significant in the paper. Papers that have a simple 'free-text' reference to the key term will not be identified using the subject headings as search terms and this can significantly affect your search, especially if your key terms are only a minor focus of a paper but of significant interest to you! Furthermore, searching is often complicated by the imaginative use of clever titles, which can obscure the exact content of papers (Hawker et al. 2002).

Ideally, you should combine the controlled search and free-text search and remove the duplicates that you get. This is the conclusion reached by DeMars and Perruso (2022), who studied the effectiveness of the two approaches. It is advisable to run different searches using different terms and compare the results you get from each one. This will demonstrate that you are taking a thoughtful and reflective approach to your search strategy.

Whichever approach you take, or decide to combine the two, you need to work out a strategy using the key terms and synonyms you have identified. We discuss how you can do this using the Boolean operators below.

Use of Boolean operators

- AND searches for two terms together and hence limits the search
- OR searches for either of two terms and hence widens the search
- NOT excludes the term from a search. Many experts recommend caution when using the NOT command in case you omit potentially relevant papers.

The important point here is to beware of using too many ANDs in a search as you might limit your search far too much. It is usually more effective to have a longer list of references and to search through them yourself than to limit your search extensively through use of Boolean operators.

Truncation

Most databases have the * (or equivalent) facility, which enables you to place the * at the end of the main stem of the word you are searching for. This will then seek out all the possible endings of the word. A note of caution here though: if you truncate a word too early, for example car* instead of care, you will get many irrelevant hits. Car* is a truncation for car, career, cart, carousel and so on (Table 4.5).

Search limiters

In addition to limiting your search to the key term in the title, abstract or full text of a paper, there are other limitations you can put on a search, including date, language, research type, human or animal, and many others. Careful judgement is needed to assess the relevance of each limiter to your review and it is unwise to restrict your search too much and risk omitting relevant literature. You will find that each database is different, and careful scrutiny of the workings of each is required to find similar limiters in different databases.

Table 4.5 Example of Boolean operators and truncation

Literature review question: 'What effect does shift length have on the delivery of nursing care?'

Nurs* OR Nurse performance OR Nursing care AND Shift pattern* OR Safe staffing OR Rota OR shift

Inclusion and exclusion criteria

Most researchers would agree that even with a well-formulated literature review question, clear inclusion and exclusion criteria are useful to guide the identification and selection of literature. Inclusion criteria allow you to specify the remit of your project, which may not be evidenced in the research question alone. They also provide a clear guide for what you are looking for when you search for literature.

Some inclusion criteria will relate to the type of research and other evidence you need to include. For example, many Cochrane reviews of the effectiveness of interventions state that RCTs will be included and all other research excluded. Other studies might state that only qualitative studies will be included. You need to consider whether country of origin of the study is relevant to your research question – for example, whether there are cultural factors in research that make international studies more or less relevant. You can set limits in most search engines to exclude some of the papers upfront.

Other inclusion criteria will be guided by pragmatic decisions. Date of publication and country of origin of the studies can be a pragmatic approach to limiting the amount of literature included in a study but the limitations of this approach should be acknowledged. Important work might have been carried out before the arbitrary cut-off date, or relevant work undertaken in a different country that has influenced the field internationally. Pragmatic approaches to defining inclusion and exclusion criteria will be necessary to all levels of post-graduate study but you will need to justify your decisions. If you are going to introduce a cut-off date, it is useful to link it to a key policy change or change in practice, for example the introduction of a new drug.

Example

In their review of predictors and consequential factors of emotional exhaustion among social workers, Chaves-Montero et al. (2025) identified the following inclusion criteria: (1) Language criteria, (2) Low scientific quality, (3) Design criteria, (4) Population relevance, (5) Qualitative and mixed-methods studies.

An important point to remember is that research and other evidence excluded as a result of the criteria set might be used in specific sections of your literature review, for example in the introduction or discussion. It is not necessarily wasted.

Practice makes perfect

Each database will operate slightly differently and it takes time and skill to learn how to use each effectively. You may need a different strategy for each database you consult. If your library runs training courses on using databases, make sure you attend as this will assist you to make the most of your searching sessions. You will always pick up new tips even if you are familiar with database searching. The main thing to emphasize with electronic searching is that it is a skill that requires practice (Just 2012; Smith and Shurtz 2012).

You can test your searching strategies by comparing the results you get using different search terms and different limiters. If a key paper is not identified in one of your searches, you should consider why that is so. Doing 'test' searches will help you justify your approach to searching when you write up the method for your literature review. It can be useful to identify five key papers that you would expect your search to identify. If your search does not find them, then it is a good indication that you need to reconsider your search strategy.

Matching your hits with your inclusion criteria

Once you have got a list of hits, or possible relevant research and other evidence from your database searches, you need to match these up with the references which, *prima facie,* seem to fit your inclusion and exclusion criteria. This is an initial match only and we will consider this in a lot more detail in the next chapter.

Assistance from a second reviewer

At this stage, it is useful to engage the assistance of a second reviewer, who you can ask to undertake the same task of comparing the list of results/hits with your inclusion criteria. Send your second reviewer a copy of your inclusion and exclusion criteria and a copy of your results/hits, although databases often have the facility to share searches between researchers. Your second reviewer can then compare the list of results/hits with the inclusion criteria. This will enable you to assess the level of agreement between the two of you as to the initial inclusion of studies in your review. The second reviewer can be your supervisor, a fellow student or another academic member of staff. It is also important to remember that the checking and verification of papers for inclusion in your review is often required by journal editors when a paper is submitted for publication.

How many hits are too many?

This is a question that frequently arises. Ideally, a focused search should filter out most irrelevant hits but it remains a judgement call regarding how many titles and abstracts you review from a database. In principle, it is wise to err on the side of reviewing a large number of hits rather than risk overlooking or omitting relevant papers. The process of identifying relevant papers from titles and abstracts can be quicker than you might imagine. It is possible to work through many hundreds of hits in a few hours. So, considering the time spent on your project as a whole, and that searching for relevant literature is fundamental to this process, time spent on this activity is wisely invested.

It is important to bear in mind that when you are searching, you do not want to artificially limit the number of hits that you get by narrowing your search too much. While a smaller number of hits might seem more manageable, the aim of the search is to direct you to a comprehensive range of literature, and you need a comprehensive search strategy to facilitate this. If you are truly inundated with hits, for example more than a few thousand, you might consider if the focus of your research question is too broad and whether there is a way you could limit the focus of the question, while retaining the appropriate depth of literature.

Recording your search results

You need to document the process of refining down your search so that the reader of your work is satisfied that relevant papers have not been omitted on the way. The PRISMA (Preferred Reporting Items for Systematic reviews and Meta-Analyses) flow chart (Figure 4.1) has been developed to help authors of systematic reviews to report their studies in a comprehensive and transparent way, demonstrating the number of references identified and their relevance to the research question (https://www.prisma-statement.org/prisma-2020?rq=PRISMA%20statement). There is also a PRISMA checklist, which helps you to report systematic reviews.

If you are submitting your literature review as a requirement for a post-graduate award, those responsible for assessing your work may spot-check your searches, taking into consideration that database entries change frequently and databases may merge. Despite this, it should be possible for an external reader of your work to replicate the searches that you have documented.

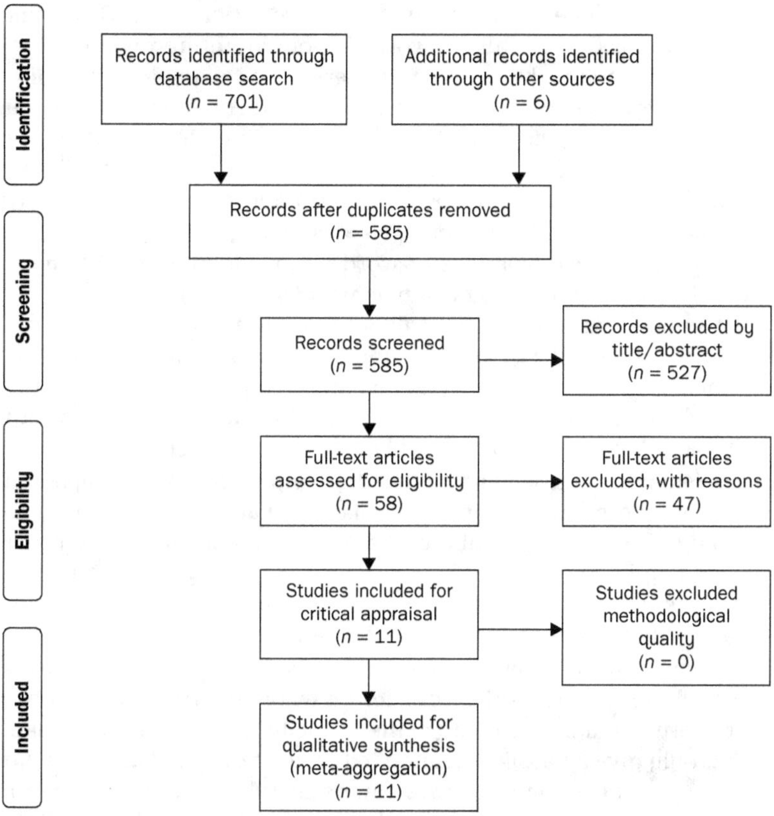

Figure 4.1 An example of a PRISMA diagram

Source: Jakimowicz et al. (2015: 26)

Common pitfalls in the searching process

Those new to searching often make the following errors when conducting their searches:

1. Using terms that are too specific or too general. You will either get far too few or far too many hits. For example, in psychology, the term 'coping' is used so widely you are likely to get directed to an unmanageable amount of hits.
2. Use of too many ANDs. Remember that AND will combine the terms you use and only identify papers that contain both terms. Therefore, if you select a search term that is very focused and combine this with

AND, you are likely to get a very narrow selection of hits. The point to remember is that not all the words in your literature review question need to be included in your search terms. For example, for the literature review question to investigate the impact of intentional rounding on patient safety, key terms would include 'intentional rounding' and 'safety' but not the term 'impact'. The term 'impact' would limit the search to papers that include this term and there may be relevant papers that do not mention impact specifically.

3. Inappropriate combinations of words (synonyms) using OR. Remember that all the terms you combine with OR must be representative of the same word. Your search will not work if you combine words that are not associated. For example, for the literature review question mentioned above, the following combinations might be made: intentional rounding OR ward round OR handover OR safety. Including safety in the same string of synonyms will make your search less effective.
4. Not enough identified and included synonyms. It is not really possible to have too many OR synonyms. Lots of ORs means that you have thought long and hard about possible synonyms and if they do not yield any hits, it won't affect your search. For example, if you limit your list of synonyms to a few popular terms, you might miss out on papers that have used an alternative term to index the paper.
5. Inappropriate key terms, or failure to state whether key terms are searched for in the title, abstract or whole text. If your key terms are very popular, searching in the whole text will refer you to papers that only give a passing mention to the key terms and you may therefore get a lot of inappropriate papers that do not focus on the topic you are researching. For example, it is good practice to undertake a search using the key terms in the whole text and then compare the hits you get when you restrict the search to the key terms in the title or abstract. Discuss this when you write up your search.
6. Inappropriate use of the truncation * command. This command allows you to search for the stem of a word so that you access all the words that begin with that stem. You need to think carefully about where the truncation command should be placed. For example, the words 'social worker' cannot be truncated down to 'social*' as this will result in far too many hits.
7. Inappropriate restriction of date and country of publication. Remember that your search should reflect your question and, as such, the restrictions you set on the search must be appropriate to the question. For example, there might be important work that has been carried out prior to the dates you set and you need to be mindful of missing significant articles that may be a little older.

Limitations of an electronic search

Most experts agree that using carefully developed key terms will maximize the success of your search strategy (Wong et al. 2004; McKibbon et al. 2006; Wilczynski et al. 2007; Papaioannou et al. 2010). However, there is also agreement that electronic database searching should not be the sole component of your overall search strategy (Wong et al. 2004; Wilczynski et al. 2007; Booth 2008; Langenhoff and Schoones 2011). Due to the limitations associated with database searching, no search will be 100 per cent effective, and a thorough search strategy requires more than a simple electronic search. This conclusion has been reached by researchers who have cross-referenced the results of electronic searching with literature identified in other ways and found that relevant pieces of research were not identified by the electronic searches. For example, Betrán et al. (2005) found that only 80 per cent of studies in their review were identified through a database search, while Mattioli et al. (2012) concluded that although good search terms made their database search more accurate, supplementary searching methods identified more literature. Developing your search to incorporate additional searching techniques will distinguish your search strategy and give your readers confidence that you have accessed a broad range of literature. This is particularly the case for topics that are difficult to search for and where your key terms are not included in the title or abstract of a paper. It is also important where your topic crosses into more than one discipline and includes policies.

Additional search strategies

The following additional search strategies have been identified and can be considered as supplementary to your electronic database searches.

Additional searching strategies are not 'haphazard' if they are combined with an electronic search. Using these strategies would only be haphazard if they were the *only* means of searching for literature. This includes judicious use of artificial intelligence. It is possible to search via AI platforms but *only* as a supplementary measure.

Berry picking

Berry picking is usually adopted as part of an expansive literature search (Bates 1989; Barroso et al. 2003; Finfgeld-Connett and Johnson 2013), although it could be argued that the approach can be used to enhance any literature search strategy. Berry picking is an ever-changing search for literature in which the researcher 'meander[s] through the bushes, looking for clumps of berries ... the searcher wanders through the information forest, changing directions as needed to follow up on various leads and shifts in thinking' (Bates 1989, cited in Barosso et al. 2003: 157). Thus, berry picking is not a linear process but one that cannot always be well mapped, involving many twists and turns along the way. The advantage of this approach is that the berry picker (or literature reviewer) can seek out good sources of 'berries' and then search around similar areas where good sources of berries have been found. Peoples et al. (2011) argue that it is not always possible to accurately define and recall the search process and that often one paper will lead to a cluster of useful papers, and that the process of achieving this may be difficult to capture. The search strategy cannot always be mapped from the outset and the way concepts are identified may defy simple reporting. Researchers may also find it hard to remember which route they actually took.

Citation tracking

If you look up a paper in certain search engines, you can see who else has cited that paper. Useful tools for this are Web of Science and Google Scholar. On Google Scholar, in the bottom right, you will see a link to cited papers. These papers may be relevant to your review and so a quick assessment of the titles will help you to identify additional papers. This means that you are also less likely to miss more recent papers.

Searching the reference lists of included papers

Searching the reference lists of papers already identified is a good approach to identifying papers that might have been missed through an electronic search. When you find papers this way, it is useful to track back and see why they were missed by your electronic search. This might give you further ideas about relevant search terms you may have missed.

Hand-searching relevant journals

Hand-searching the contents pages of relevant journals is another common approach to identifying papers that might have been missed during an electronic search. You can search either the contents page, or the complete issue of the journal page by page. Again, you might track back and consider why any papers that you find this way were not identified in your electronic search. You can then amend your search strategy to include key terms that have been identified that were not apparent previously.

Author searching

There are likely to be some key authors and researchers who have published in your area. Thus an additional search can be done using the electronic databases in which you search under the authors' names rather than using key terms. This way, you may identify additional research or other evidence published in your field of study.

Using automatic targeting systems

Citrome et al. (2009) discuss services that alert you to relevant articles and send you those articles direct via electronic communication. Lots of journals and databases have 'alerts' lists. For example, the NCBI (National Centre for Biotechnology Information) has a customized profile in which you store key terms. These are searched for you on a regular basis. Really Simple Syndication (RSS) feeds provide automatic feeds of relevant information. You can also formulate a question and put it online and the papers are directed to you (Citrome et al. 2009).

Locating unpublished literature, including theses and dissertations, monographs, reports and conference abstracts

Depending on the scope of your literature review, these additional search strategies are useful for identifying unpublished material that might lead you to other significant sources. In addition, contacting the authors of papers that are widely cited in your topic area might lead you to further sources of useful research or other evidence (Flemming et al. 2013).

Books and book chapters

Books and book chapters are not only likely to be useful for background reading for your project but may also be a rich source for the presentation and discussion of theories and concepts that may be related to your work.

Cessation of searching

No matter the approach you adopt to literature searching, it is difficult to know when to stop searching. In some approaches, for example for Cochrane systematic reviews with meta-analysis, searching ends once the searching protocol has been completed. For other reviews, cessation of searching is a judgement call as it is never possible to know with any certainty whether all the literature has been located or whether further literature could be found that would contribute significantly to the review and has been missed by a premature end to the searching (Barroso et al. 2003; Booth 2010). However, the approach that you take to the review will provide you with a rationale to end the search. For a comprehensive search, the searching typically ends when all the planned searches have been carried out. For anyone doing a purposive or selective search, searching typically ends when no new themes are identified in the literature. There might also be limitations due to the scale of the project, such as time or other resource constraints.

Practicalities for conducting a thorough search

Consider the use of software (for example, Endnote) in which you can save references, abstracts and PDFs. There are also versions that allow you to share references. You can import findings from your searches straight into these reference management systems, although we would recommend limiting your imports to potentially relevant papers to prevent overloading the system. Even citation tracking searches can be entered simply if you set up Google Scholar to allow for 'one click' importing into your reference management system. There are many other alternatives that can be shared. The learning technologist at your academic institution or your academic librarian will be able to advise you on the various options available.

Searching for related research and other evidence if there is minimal literature

If your search remains somewhat limited and you have not identified sufficient research or other evidence to address your research question, you can consider searching for literature that addresses a parallel area. The specific focus you wish to address might not have been researched in your area but might have been explored in relation to a related area – for example, with another population or client group, with a different condition or situation, and so on. It is then possible to draw parallels from the identified literature to address your own literature review question.

In summary

The literature you include in your review is determined by your review question. This is guided by your inclusion and exclusion criteria. Unless you have a good reason not to, we recommend that you undertake a comprehensive search for research and other evidence that meets your inclusion and exclusion criteria. You need to consider that you may have more than one review question and that each will need separate inclusion and exclusion criteria and hence a separate search. A more selective search might be appropriate for additional searches for theoretical or methodological aspects of your review, depending on the findings of your main search.

Searching is a time-consuming process and you need to adopt a clear strategy that will direct you to the appropriate research and other evidence to include in your review. This strategy will include searching subject-specific electronic databases in addition to supplementary strategies such as hand-searching journals, author searching, citation searching and wider searches. If you get too many hits, do not artificially reduce them by limiting your search inappropriately, but you may need to reconsider the focus of your search. It is important that you document your search so that others could replicate it if required and so it demonstrates that you have been rigorous in your searching. There is a lot of software that enables you to search, share and store your references. You may be asked to account for your search strategy in an oral examination.

Key points

- You need to undertake a comprehensive search for each question you have identified in your review
- Artificial intelligence cannot currently do this for you: the review process is too nuanced
- You may supplement this search with additional searching in order to develop your understanding of theories and methods that may be relevant to your project

- You need to be able to justify which aspects of your search need to be fully comprehensive and when a more selective search is appropriate
- Decide on a strategy for your searching, including electronic database searching and additional methods
- Reconsider your searching approach if you get too many or too few hits
- Consider software that enables you to search, share results and store your data
- Ensure this strategy is fully documented within your review.

5

Selection of relevant papers and data extraction

In this chapter, we will discuss:

- *How you can identify relevant papers for your review*
- *How you can extract and summarize the data that is relevant to your review*
- *How data extraction forms assist with this process*
- *How data extraction forms can be adapted for your individual project.*

At this stage, you have completed appropriate searches for your literature review as discussed in Chapter 4, and will have identified papers that potentially you could include in your review. This will usually include empirical research in addition to the relevant discussion of theoretical perspectives and methodological issues where appropriate. The next step is to identify what is relevant for inclusion in your review. In order to make your review as systematic as possible, there are steps you can follow to ensure this is a rigorous process. This will prevent your review from becoming an 'ad hoc' collection of studies and transform it into one that is clearly and logically thought through and defendable in the written report or oral examination.

This chapter relates most closely to your empirical review, for which you have a clear research question and inclusion and exclusion criteria to guide you. This can be either for a standalone review or one that is a prerequisite for a larger empirical study. Where you have done additional searches for theoretical and methodological papers to enhance your discussion of theories and methods you have used, your use of data extraction methods may be less extensive.

Selection of possible papers from titles and abstracts

The first step in the selection of papers is to read through the titles and identify those that *appear* to meet your inclusion criteria, which we discussed in Chapter 4.

You might find that the results of some studies are reported in more than one paper. Sometimes different aspects of studies are reported in different papers. This is referred to as 'salami slicing', where researchers understandably seek to maximize the number of possible publications from a study. This practice can also be complicated when researchers in a team rotate authorship of papers that refer to different aspects of their study. A little 'detective work' can usually enable you to determine whether the study described in a paper is the same as that referred to in another paper; for example, if the sample size and location of the study are the same, this might indicate that the authors are reporting the same study in different papers. If it is still unclear, you can contact the authors directly to check. Another potential area for confusion is studies that are initially published as pilot studies or protocol papers and then subsequently published in full after the main study is completed. Usually, only the fully completed study will be useful for your literature review, although if the pilot study has been published in its own right, rather than its data incorporated into a later study, then it might be eligible for inclusion in the review.

The importance of documenting your method should be flagged up again here. As with all sections of a literature review, it is useful to document what you have done at all stages. This helps to keep the review transparent and rigorous but, more importantly, it allows you to keep a record of what you have done so that you do not repeat tasks unnecessarily, in what can be a complicated process.

It is recommended to start to document the process of selecting papers using a flow chart, as illustrated in Chapter 4. This will include information about how many hits you had from all of the searches, and how you reduced this number by scanning the titles of papers. It is also important to document how many duplicate references to the same paper you found on different databases. We have already discussed how it is useful to ask a second person to assist you in this task.

Reviewing the title of each paper alone might not be sufficient to enable you to decide about its relevance to your project and you may want to check the abstract too. This can be done as either a 'one-stage' or 'two-stage' process. You may decide to look at abstracts of potential papers as you find the titles, or you may prefer to check titles first and then check the abstracts in a separate check. Not all the databases you use will give you access to an abstract and you may have to access the full paper to get it. Whichever approach you decide to take, it is important to keep a record of abstracts that you have and have not seen, as it is easy to lose track.

Access to the full text of the paper: hard copy or e-copy

Once you have identified any relevant papers from their titles and abstracts, you need to clarify whether they fully meet the inclusion criteria you have identified and hence whether or not they should be included in your literature review.

In order to do this, you need to obtain the full-text version or e-copy of the full paper so that further consideration of the relevance and the quality of the paper can be made. If you have not yet checked the abstract, you need to review the abstract in the first instance, to determine whether the paper is relevant.

Getting to know your papers

Once you have undertaken an initial check of full papers, read each thoroughly. This might sound obvious, but understanding each paper is key to determining its relevance and there are no shortcuts you can take. Artificial intelligence might provide a summary for you but it will not capture the details that you need to fully understand each paper. It is the literature reviewer's equivalent to the qualitative researcher 'getting immersed in the data'. It is not possible to analyse your research and other evidence without a thorough knowledge of each paper. This includes knowing the research designs of the papers you are using. As you read a paper, you may find that the research design is not the one you are interested in for your review. For example, you might be looking for RCTs only and the research design you have is quasi-experimental. You might find that the intervention used in one paper is different from that used in another one and you will need to make a judgement as to its relevance to your review. For example, if you are reviewing the effectiveness of music therapy in relieving the symptoms of depression in people with dementia, you will need to consider whether music therapy encompasses participation in music-making in addition to listening to music. Alternatively, you might find that the population is not relevant for your review. The populations included within a paper might be diverse, or several similar populations may be included within one study. If you are only interested in one sub-population, you will need to consider whether you can access data about the population you are interested in without 'contaminating' your data with information from a population that you are not interested in. These are judgements that you need to make.

Determining the relevance of the paper to your literature review

Once you have got to know your papers well, the next step is to consider the relevance of each paper to your review. We suggest that you do this thoroughly in the first instance so that only papers that are considered relevant are then critically appraised.

Screening the full paper against your inclusion and exclusion criteria

The first step in identifying relevant papers is to consider the full version of each paper against your inclusion and exclusion criteria. You have already done this with the title and abstract but you now need to consider each paper in full. It is useful to keep a record of this so that you can refer back to it when you write up your method of searching and identification of literature.

A simple inclusion/exclusion criteria tool to facilitate the identification of relevant papers is shown in Table 5.1. If you use a form such as this you can demonstrate that you have followed a process for assessing whether the paper is relevant to your review.

At this stage, the focus of each paper is the key criterion for inclusion and a more detailed examination of included papers would follow. When you use a summary sheet to assess papers for inclusion and exclusion, a paper trail is created to which you can return rather than trawling through each paper again.

Table 5.1 Example of a checklist for checking your paper against inclusion and exclusion criteria

Inclusion criteria – specifically designed for your review (answers to all questions should be **yes**)

Example criteria:

- Is the study population over 16 years old?
- Does the study population have symptomatic pleural effusion from an underlying malignant process?
- Does the study compare drug treatments for pleural effusion via the intra-pleural route?
- Is the trial an RCT or a randomized crossover trial?

Exclusion criteria – specifically designed for your review (answers to all questions should be **no**)

- Does the study include patients with both malignant and non-malignant disease with no clear distinction between the groups in the results?
- Is the study evaluating the effect of a drug administered via a method other than the intra-pleural route?
- Does the study include effusions in a number of different body cavities (for example, peritoneum, pericardium), with no distinction between the groups in the results section?

On this section of the screening form, you are likely to include the following information:

- Identification of paper, author(s) and year of publication
- Name of person completing the data extraction if part of a larger study
- Date of data extraction
- Inclusion and exclusion criteria for your literature review.

It should be emphasized that these inclusion and exclusion criteria are those developed by you for your own review. It can be useful to add a table and a check box to highlight whether the paper has met your inclusion and exclusion criteria.

Assistance from a second reviewer

The decision to include or exclude may not be easy to make and it might be useful to seek the assistance of a second reviewer at this point. You can ask them to help you identify relevant articles from the full paper, rather than just the title or abstract. This is a useful process in its own right but can be especially useful if you are unsure about the inclusion of a paper; any uncertainty can be settled by reaching a consensus with the second reviewer. Many journals require the input from a second or third reviewer if you submit your paper for publication.

Example of a checklist for inclusion and exclusion criteria

In the example given in Table 5.1, the inclusion and exclusion criteria are for a literature review that was conducted as part of a PhD study to explore the effectiveness of treatment in the management of patients with pleural effusion due to an underlying malignancy. A malignant pleural effusion is the collection of fluid in the pleural space around the lung in a person with a malignancy. It is important to emphasize that these charts must be developed for each individual review and you should be able to defend your rationale for the inclusion and exclusion criteria you set. On the checklist that you create, remember to include a way to identify the study, the authors' names, name of reviewer, date and decision.

For this literature review of the effectiveness of interventions for the reduction of pleural effusion due to malignant disease, the focus is on effectiveness and therefore any studies that do not compare one treatment option against another or a placebo ought to be excluded, even if they are related to the management of pleural effusion and identified in a search. Therefore, only randomized controlled studies that considered the effectiveness of treatment for pleural effusion should be included. This was stated in the inclusion criteria for the study. Note that it is not always possible to identify the type of study that will be included in the review. This will depend on the question but requires consideration when you formulate your inclusion and exclusion criteria and will be reviewed when you write your data extraction form.

Once you have reviewed and selected your papers based on your inclusion and exclusion criteria, you will have an almost complete list of papers for inclusion in your review. You can now undertake a detailed assessment of each paper.

This assessment process comprises consideration of two main concepts:

- Data extraction
- Quality of the paper (critical appraisal).

We will consider data extraction in the remainder of this chapter, and critical appraisal will be discussed in Chapter 6.

Data extraction (data summary)

Data extraction is a process that enables you to extract the relevant information from the papers that are included in your study in preparation for subsequent analysis. Without a logical data extraction process, you will be faced with the task of trying to make sense of a paper without having identified the relevant aspects for your analysis. Identifying in each paper exactly what is relevant to your review will help you prepare your papers for the subsequent process of data analysis. At the time of writing, it is not possible for artificial intelligence to replicate this process with the precision and judgement required.

Data extraction form (data summary form)

A data extraction form (or data summary sheet) is a tool that helps you to manage and process your data (the literature), which will help you select the papers you need for your review and ultimately will help you to write up your literature review. The data extraction (or data summary) sheet will help you to summarize the key points about a paper and, if this is done thoroughly, can help you identify key aspects of that paper that are relevant to your research question, thus saving you from having to re-read it each time you want to check a particular detail.

In the data extraction form, you can collect key data from the papers, which will help you in three ways:

1. To confirm that the paper is relevant for your review
2. To focus your thoughts and ideas about the paper
3. To provide a summary document about the paper.

As with the initial checklist used to identify papers according to the inclusion and exclusion criteria, we suggest that you develop a data extraction sheet that is specific to the needs of your review.

How you use the data extraction sheet will depend on your study question and you will develop one in line with your individual study. Usually, it is possible to adapt a data extraction sheet from another project rather than creating your own from scratch. However, your data extraction form will be unique to your individual literature review. There are common features to the form that are likely to be relevant to all studies. A completed data extraction tool is shown in the Appendix.

When devising your data extraction sheet, you need to focus on what is important for your study, otherwise the data extraction will not be 'fit for purpose' and you will find that you need to keep returning to the original papers. However, for some in-depth qualitative studies, it might not be possible to capture the main aspects of a study upon first reading and you will find that you need to consult the original paper many times before you are confident that you have summarized it appropriately on the data extraction sheet.

The detail with which you undertake this stage will depend on the role of the literature review within your project and the scale of your project. If your literature review is a prerequisite to an empirical study at MSc level, you will have less scope to develop this aspect of your review than if it is a standalone review or a prerequisite to an empirical study for a PhD.

You may decide to complete a data extraction sheet for each potential paper that you have identified. A note of caution, however: if you have a particularly large number of 'possible' papers, it is unlikely you will be able to complete a data extraction sheet for each one. You will not know at this stage which papers will be included in your final literature review.

Below we provide two examples of data extraction forms together with some of the principles used to develop them. The first example (Table 5.2) is a quantitative form and the second one (Table 5.3) a qualitative form. We have included a completed data extraction form in the Appendix.

Example of a data extraction form for a systematic review of randomized controlled trials

You can see from our first example (Table 5.2) that a carefully constructed data extraction form will enable you to draw out very detailed information about the study. It is not possible to know in advance which data you extract will be used in your final analysis; some papers might contain minimal reference to the sort of information you are interested in but you won't know this until you have read each paper in turn. This means, of course, that you will extract a lot of data that you will never use in your analysis. Once you have established the type(s) of study design (if appropriate), you need to identify which details about that study design you need to report. For the study in Table 5.2, the

Table 5.2 Data extraction form for a systematic review of randomized controlled trials

Details about the study			
Country or countries			
Start of recruitment			
End of recruitment			
Intended duration of follow-up for each patient (months) – please state maximum			
Number of recruiting centres			
If >1 recruiting centres, is the trial cluster randomized? (Yes/No/NA)			
Type of report (F = full text; A = abstract; U = unpublished)			
Language			
What is the study evaluating? (A = pleurodesis agent; B = mode of admin of pleurodesis; C = other method to optimize pleurodesis; D = IPC)			
Details of the intervention			
Common treatment for all groups (therefore not under comparison)			
Group	1	2	3
Description of intervention			
Dose			
Number of doses given and frequency			
Mode of administration			
Number of patients randomized			
Number lost to follow-up and reasons			
Which group was used as the control? (tick one)			
How did you decide which was the control group? (tick one)	Assumed by data extractor ☐ Stated in paper ☐		

researchers required information about trial design; for example, whether it was a cluster design or a simple RCT. In addition, they required information about the intervention; with a drug trial, this is about drug dose and frequency, but with another form of intervention, such as a service-delivery model, the intervention needs to be clearly documented. You also need to consider how the success, or not, of the intervention was defined and measured. It is not always clearly stated in a paper how an outcome has been measured, and you might consider contacting the authors if this is the case.

In this literature review, the primary outcome might be described as the complete removal of fluid, as identified on X-ray or by the absence of symptomatic signs of fluid. A few research papers, especially those published some time ago, might not provide any detailed information on this and merely report a successful drainage of fluid without an accompanying definition. Much of this information needs to be assessed and clarification sought from the authors if possible. The primary outcome measure from your review may be different from the primary outcome of the paper as it may be a secondary outcome measure. You will have decided upon your primary outcome for the review but also some secondary outcome measures and adverse event reporting.

If you are going to undertake a meta-analysis, you need to decide what will be considered 'good enough' results for inclusion in your analysis. Absolute values are then recorded according to the number randomized in each arm, numbers analysed in each arm and those lost to follow-up. This is important so as to assess for bias in the study. For more details on extracting data for RCTs, see the *Cochrane Handbook for Systematic Reviews of Interventions* (Higgins et al. 2024). For before-and-after study designs, and quasi-experimental or controlled studies, similar data will be collected.

Data extraction form for qualitative or mixed-methods studies

Data extraction forms for qualitative and mixed-methods studies are slightly different, as the process of analysing literature data tends to be more iterative and less of a 'one-off' event. The way in which you develop your data extraction form for qualitative research papers will depend on the approach you take to your analysis. If there is a large body of work that has already been undertaken in your field of study, your analysis of the literature can be undertaken deductively. In this case, it is possible to pre-specify themes from the existing body of literature that will be searched for in the different papers that make up your review. Anyone undertaking a framework analysis, which we discuss in Chapter 7, will use this approach. In this case, you can tailor your data extraction form to pre-specify the areas of interest you are searching for. More usually, however, data analysis is inductive, where the reviewers retain an open stance to the literature and identify themes as they arise from the papers rather than imposing a pre-established framework. In this case, it is not possible to pre-state concepts in a data extraction sheet, as you will not be aware of what these concepts are until you have read the research. However, you can develop this form so that you can create a table to which you can extract the themes that arise in your data straight away. Remember, tables can be used to describe your data and highlight themes but the craft of your synthesis will come in how you discuss and synthesize the findings from the tables. We will discuss this further in Chapter 7.

As with all research, you need to read and re-read each paper to ensure that you have a thorough understanding of what it is about, and you need to ensure that you stay close to the data at all times. What, at first glance, may seem to be an appropriate interpretation of a paper might be revised on later reading and in comparison with other papers, when your understanding of the research area has developed.

We provide an example of a data extraction form for a qualitative or mixed-methods systematic review in Table 5.3, together with some of the principles used to develop the form. The purpose of this literature review was to explore the perceptions of services by people experiencing a life-limiting illness. As with the quantitative data extraction form above, a carefully constructed form will enable you to draw out very detailed information about the study. In this study, the researchers used both qualitative and quantitative research to address their aims. Because of the broad focus of the research, data extraction had to be selective and relevant to the literature review question.

It is important to find out about the participants so that you can understand the context in which the findings or themes are discussed. It is also useful to retain as much context as possible to avoid misinterpretation of the data at the analysis stage. It is useful to extract as much of this information as possible.

In this study, the methods used to explore users' perception were varied. You need to record the approach taken in the study, including data collection and analysis approaches. The data extraction table needs to be able to accommodate a variety of methods rather than just having

Table 5.3 Data extraction form for a qualitative or mixed-methods systematic review

		Details about the study			
Author, country, score	**Research question or aim of study**	**Participants**	**Method**	**Palliative care team**	**Key themes**
Dharmasena and Forbes (2001), UK, 25	Will doctors refer non-cancer patients to palliative care?	78 consultants	Postal survey, 8 items. Analysis not described	Not described	Model of care; professional onus; expertise and trust; skill building vs. deskilling
Salomon et al. (2001), France, 30	To describe the current management of terminally ill patients from care providers' viewpoint	31 physicians, 16 nurses	Structured, self-administered, 33-item survey. SPSS (statistical package for the social sciences) used for analysis	Physician, nurse, psychologist	Model of care; skill building vs. deskilling; specialist palliative care operations
Carter et al. (2002), New Zealand, 29	To determine health professionals' perception of the service's impact on patients, families and staff, and areas that need improvement	127 doctors, 242 nurses, 11 social workers	Postal survey, 5-point Likert scale and yes/no questions. EPI6 used for analysis	Full-time nurse, part-time physician	Model of care; skill building vs deskilling; specialist palliative care operations

tick boxes. This is especially important for qualitative methods, where the approaches used are often diverse and might have been adapted to suit the needs of the study.

You need to identify the key themes that arise in relation to your review question. You could choose to provide these in detail on the data extraction form or you might do so in another table. Sometimes the key themes that have been identified by the researchers in their analysis of their data will be relevant to your review but this depends on your review question. You might identify alternative themes or re-name the themes used in the original paper.

Sample data extraction for non-research evidence

Depending on your inclusion and exclusion criteria, you may have included non-research papers in your review. If you have done so, you will need to extract data from these in a similar way to the research papers included in the review. As with all papers, it is important to extract only the data that are relevant to answering your review question.

You might find it useful to develop a data extraction form for evidence other than the research papers that you include in your review (Table 5.4). The same principles apply; the purpose of the data extraction form is to provide clarity and a standardized approach to the evidence you have so that you can use it in your subsequent analysis.

Pilot testing the data extraction forms

Once you have developed the full data extraction form, you are ready to begin in earnest. At this point, we suggest that you identify two papers that you are fairly confident will be included in your review. You can use these to model or test out your data extraction form.

Table 5.4 Data extraction form for non-research

Author (year) country	Type of evidence	Type of arguments	Main outcomes
Who wrote the paper, when and where?	Is the evidence discussion or a more developed theory?	How are the arguments expressed?	What are the main messages?

The data extraction form will usually revisit the initial inclusion and exclusion criteria. This is because when a paper is examined in more detail, you might then decide to exclude it from your review. It is also possible that some papers might have been rejected inappropriately during initial data extraction, which is why you need to remain open to the possibility of returning to the original papers at any stage of your literature review.

Once you have tested out your data extraction form, we suggest that you and a colleague, or member of the review team if you have one, review up to five papers independently of each other. You can then come together to see if you have completed the forms in similar ways. It may be that your second reviewer has interpreted some of your data extraction questions in a different way. Or you may have failed to record some vital pieces of information that you didn't intend collecting initially, such as length of hospital stay, cost or mortality data. At this point, you can add further sections to your form to add clarity.

At the end of all this, you should have a data extraction form that is pilot tested and that you are confident will help you to summarize the data from the literature you intend to include in your review. We suggest that you complete a data extraction form for each study that you have identified as potentially relevant for your review and that you document this when you write up your method section of your thesis.

In summary

Once you have identified which papers meet your inclusion and exclusion criteria, the next step is to read the papers thoroughly and extract the details of those that are relevant for your review. This is usually done with your empirical literature but the process can be useful when you are reviewing theories and concepts in your review. This process is often referred to as data extraction, and the purpose is to organize and standardize the data so that you can see clearly how they relate to your review question. Data extraction is concerned with exploring the detailed results from a study you are intending to include in your literature review. The data extraction process helps you to process the results of the research or other evidence you have and to clarify your understanding of a paper. It is useful to develop a data extraction sheet so that you can summarize the results of the papers onto one form. This serves two purposes: it provides clarity about the papers and it prevents you from having to refer back to the original studies. Data extraction is different from critical appraisal, which we will explore in the next chapter.

Key points

- Papers you have identified as possible for selection in your review need to be compared against your inclusion and exclusion criteria
- Papers that meet your inclusion criteria need to be carefully considered to check they are relevant to your review
- In order to focus on the detail of the included papers, data extraction sheets should be developed
- Data extraction is a useful way to prepare your papers for subsequent data analysis
- These need to be specific to the individual study but can be adapted from other studies
- Data extraction is a separate process from critical appraisal.

6

Critical appraisal of the literature

In this chapter, we will discuss:

- *The importance of identifying the strengths and weaknesses of the papers you include*
- *Considerations to make when appraising quantitative and qualitative research*
- *Different tools that might assist with the process of critical appraisal*
- *The importance of using critical appraisal when you analyse and synthesize the papers.*

Once you have read all of the papers that are relevant for your review and undertaken a data extraction process where appropriate, the next stage is critical appraisal of the papers.

What is critical appraisal?

Critical appraisal is the process of carefully and systematically assessing the quality of the literature, in which you have to judge its trustworthiness and value in a particular context. In quantitative research, this is often referred to as identifying bias (Smith and Noble 2025). It is important to consider how the research has been conducted and the strengths and weaknesses of the other evidence you are considering for inclusion in your review, because you need to make a judgement about the quality of the evidence and hence the weight it should command when you analyse and synthesize the papers; that is, you will give greater emphasis to the stronger studies in your review. Elsewhere, Aveyard et al. (2026) provide a critical appraisal of 10 different research papers, demonstrating what to look for when you are reading a research paper. Incorporating poorly designed studies, or to give them the same weight as a stronger study, can be misleading and will affect the results of your review. Therefore, you need to consider how to deal with the stronger and weaker studies in your review.

Many students and researchers are familiar with the concept of critical appraisal. A common error, however, is to undertake a critical appraisal of the studies but then fail to make use of the critical appraisal in the subsequent analysis and synthesis of literature. Critical appraisal is only useful if you use it in your analysis. We will discuss this in Chapter 7.

An important point to make about critical appraisal is that it is not an end in itself. It is not a standalone component of a review that needs to be done and then promptly dismissed. Critical appraisal needs to be incorporated into your data analysis and synthesis, and you must take into account the impact of both the stronger and weaker studies when drawing conclusions. This requires a value judgement, which you will need to justify when you consider your analysis and synthesis of your literature (discussed in Chapter 7) and when you write up your literature review (discussed in Chapter 8).

The following example illustrates how critical appraisal of studies that you consider for inclusion in your review can have a significant impact on the results of the review. In this example, omitting studies that had been less well conducted dramatically changed the outcome of the systematic review.

Inclusion and exclusion of studies in a literature review according to quality assessment

The following is a classic example of the difference that the inclusion or exclusion of certain studies can make to the findings of a systematic review. In 2011, Gotzsche and Nielsen published a systematic review in which they had analysed the effectiveness of mammography in preventing mortality from breast cancer. The authors surveyed a wide range of studies, including those with weaker methods, that compared the mortality rate of women who had had a mammography for the early detection of breast cancer with those who had not. The researchers concluded that the benefit of mammography in preventing breast cancer deaths was marginal. Because of the controversy this study provoked, a second systematic review was undertaken. In the second review (Marmot et al. 2012), the researchers made different decisions about the inclusion of older, less well-conducted studies and included only those studies that they judged to have used stronger methods. Their review came to a different conclusion. By excluding the weaker studies, Marmot et al. (2012) found that those women who underwent mammography breast screening had an approximately 20 per cent lower risk of mortality from breast cancer.

Thus, the inclusion of methodologically stronger and weaker studies in your review can have a major impact on the outcome. Some reviews exclude weaker studies while others include them but give them less weight in the analysis. Either way, the importance of critical appraisal and the role it plays in your review is evident, something that has been discussed in depth by Carroll et al. (2012). This illustrates the importance of appraising the strengths and weaknesses of papers in the literature you have and how you will treat the stronger and weaker studies in your subsequent analysis and synthesis.

Assessing quality and risk of bias

Given the importance of undertaking a quality assessment of the research and other evidence you include in your review, the next question is how this should be done. While there is agreement that considerations of quality must be made, the question of what constitutes quality is not so easy to resolve. Quality assessment both for qualitative and quantitative research and for other evidence can be a complex process and we discuss this below. It is because of the continuing debate about quality assessment that we advise you to undertake your quality assessment only once you have confirmed that the research or other evidence is relevant for your review and you have completed the data extraction process. In this way, you critically appraise only the papers that you intend to use within your review and do not consider the quality of literature that may not be relevant to your review. Quality assessment is then undertaken once you have established that a piece of research or other evidence is relevant to your review.

The process of critical appraisal does not necessarily require the use of a tool, but tools can be useful and we will discuss this later in the chapter. The appraisal process is similar regardless of the type of analysis you undertake. Critical appraisal is the process of identifying how well the research has been conducted.

Quality standards in quantitative studies

In quantitative research methods, there is a long tradition of developing and testing research methods so that we now know the best ways of conducting research. In quantitative research, there is homogeneity of fundamental principles, including the nature of truth and reality, such that many different factors can lead to potential bias in a study. Studies are assessed according to these different areas of potential risk, and an overall assessment of the risk of bias can be considered to be high, unclear or low.

For example, Sibbald and Roland (1998) described the process of undertaking an RCT and the essential steps involved:

- There is random allocation
- Participants and clinicians are unaware of treatment allocation if possible
- Intervention groups are managed in the same way as the control group
- Participants are analysed in the group they were allocated to
- Analysis is focused on estimating the difference in size in predetermined criteria.

Subsequently, there has been much discussion, and some research has been undertaken into determining optimum ways to carry out the randomization process: for example, with the use of a truly random method such as a computer program, or an approach that conceals any randomization list so that the clinical team cannot second-guess which group the next participant will be allocated to (Schulz and Grimes 2002; Akoberg 2005).

Further information on risk of bias can be found in the Cochrane Collaboration Handbook (Higgins et al. 2024). The Cochrane Collaboration has developed a bias assessment tool (Higgins et al. 2024) for the potential sources of bias identified above.

In questionnaire design, to take another example, there are generally agreed principles regarding rigour in the development and administration of the questionnaire. These are discussed by Leung (2001) in a linked Cochrane resource. The keys areas to consider in a questionnaire study are:

- The design of the questionnaire
- The testing of the questionnaire
- The administration of the questionnaire
- The sample that will complete the questionnaire.

When the key features of a research design are established, you can use them as a benchmark against which you can compare the studies you identify and draw a conclusion about the quality of the research you have. For example, you might decide to include only questionnaires that contain a particular outcome measure based upon psychometric properties, and those tested more robustly would be included over others or given more weight.

In addition to knowledge and understanding of quantitative research methods, various statements and checklists have also been put in place to standardize approaches to quality. For example, the CONSORT statement, which was originally developed as a tool to enhance quality in the publication of RCTs, can also be used as a tool to measure the quality of RCTs (Tong et al. 2007). There are also many critical appraisal tools that focus on the assessment of quality of quantitative studies, which we will describe later in the chapter.

Quality standards in qualitative studies

In qualitative research, as in quantitative methods, there is continued research and debate about optimal methods. However, because there is more heterogeneity in the methods used, agreement about quality is more elusive. The difficulty of using predetermined quality standards for qualitative research and avoiding ritualistic approaches has been addressed by many researchers (Cleary et al. 2014). This is due to the diversity of qualitative approaches that have been developed in response to the need to research a wide range of research questions. Qualitative approaches need to be flexible and creative enough to meet the methodological demands of the study. For example, Wiles et al. (2011) identified 57 qualitative studies published between 2000 and 2009 that claimed to have developed innovative approaches in response to the individual needs of the qualitative designs. Shin et al. (2009) also identified a wide range of methods and strategies incorporated into what they described as qualitative research. However, while qualitative research designs need to be flexible, they must also retain academic rigour. Whittemore et al. argue that 'creativity must be preserved within qualitative research but not at the expense of the quality of the science' (2001: 526). Debate exists as to what constitutes reasonable deviation from an established approach in response to one's needs (Aveyard and Neale 2009). Such diversity requires a broad range of quality indicators in qualitative research.

Assessment of quality in qualitative research: flexible guidelines and transparency

Lincoln and Guba (1985) argue that qualitative research should be assessed in terms of credibility, transferability, dependability and confirmability, and suggest that these are more appropriate for assessing quality than the more traditional terms 'validity' and 'reliability', which are widely used within quantitative research. Lincoln and Guba (1985) also argue that all qualitative research should have a 'truth value' based on strategies that represent the hallmark of good qualitative research, such as keeping an accurate account of the research process and transparency in the data analysis process, rather than specifications about the process of conducting the research per se. This seminal work set a precedent for openness and transparency in the reporting of qualitative studies.

Walsh and Downe (2006) also argue that transparency and openness are the quality standards for qualitative research. In their literature review of the way in which quality is assessed in qualitative studies, the authors identified eight existing checklists and frameworks. From their analysis of these checklists and frameworks, they suggest that the assessment of qualitative research should incorporate a method that is consistent with the intent of the research, researcher reflexivity, ethical dimensions, a literature review and an analytical approach.

Spencer et al. (2003) identified four central principles for guiding the assessment of qualitative research:

- Contributes to our understanding
- Defensible in design
- Rigorous in conduct
- Transparent and systematic.

These principles focus on description and rationale for the approaches followed rather than prescription of approaches, although they do indicate other quality issues such as that interviews should be audio recorded and context of data should be preserved.

In their paper 'Consolidated criteria for the reporting of qualitative research', Tong et al. (2007) emphasized the importance within qualitative research of discussion of the research team and reflexivity, the study design, and analysis and findings.

In their review of the quality assessment of qualitative studies for research into adapted physical activity, Zitomer and Goodwin (2014) identified various approaches to the assessment of quality in 56 papers and argued for a set of 'flexible guidelines' rather than rigid criteria to guide the assessment of qualitative research. They identified the following concepts relevant to the assessment of qualitative research: credibility, resonance, significant contribution, ethics and coherence.

The QARI tool for assessing qualitative studies was developed by the Joanna Briggs Institute (2014) and focuses on three elements of qualitative research:

- Whether there is congruity between the philosophy, methodology, method, presentation of data and their interpretation
- Whether any bias and assumptions made are explicit
- Whether the relationship between what the participants are reported to have said and the conclusions of the study is clearly made.

These examples illustrate that the assessment of quality in qualitative studies has a clear focus on the transparency of reporting and flexibility of approaches rather than on defining specific rules for the conduct of qualitative research. Although this captures the essence of qualitative research, it falls short of definitive guidance on what a reviewer should be looking for in terms of quality indicators when considering the merits of a qualitative study.

Incorporating qualitative studies in a literature review

While the focus on flexibility and transparency allows much room for the discretion of the researcher in the development of quality in the study, it also gives the same discretion to the reviewer in considering the assessment of quality when including qualitative studies in a review. The benchmarks for quality are open to interpretation and it can be difficult for the literature reviewer to decide which studies they should include on the basis of quality. As a result, there is a difference of opinion in the research literature regarding how to judge the quality of qualitative studies and whether or not they should be excluded from a literature review on the basis of quality. One approach is to exclude studies on the basis of a predetermined quality assessment. Examples of organizations and individuals who follow this approach are the Joanna Briggs Institute (2014), Harden (2007) and Henry et al. (2020).

Another approach is to include all studies in the review, irrespective of the perceived quality. Carroll et al. (2012) have debated this in some detail and argue that the inclusion of weaker studies in a qualitative review does not significantly affect the analysis. Researchers who have followed this approach include Dixon-Woods et al. (2007), Noyes and Popay (2007), Atkins et al. (2008), Finfgeld-Connett (2014), Giles and Hall (2014), Smiddy et al. (2015), Rock et al. (2015) and Damarell et al. (2020).

Incorporating mixed-methods studies in a literature review

Assessment of quality in mixed-methods studies is focused on the way in which the components (usually qualitative and quantitative) are integrated. These components should not be viewed separately but rather as a combined whole which demonstrates how data collected from different perspectives contributes to the new knowledge developed in the research. So for example, if a survey is included in a mixed-methods research, resist the temptation to use the survey data as an end point in itself. Its use is maximised when it is viewed together with the qualitative component.

Critical appraisal tools for assessing quality

Debates about the assessment and inclusion of quality of research, especially in relation to qualitative studies, will not be resolved within the timescale of your post-graduate project, and you need to find a pragmatic approach to incorporating issues of quality. In order to assist with this, many critical appraisal tools have been developed for the assessment of research, and these can be a useful aid to determining the quality of an individual research study. In addition to critical appraisal tools for research, there are also critical appraisal tools for assessing the quality of arguments, theories, guidelines and policy. They are not an essential requirement of any post-graduate project, however, and such tools cannot be used as a substitute for your own careful consideration of the research and other evidence you use. You need to understand the methods undertaken in a study before you apply a critical appraisal tool.

The use of an appraisal tool is generally advised for anyone undertaking post-graduate study (Whiting et al. 2017); however, there are many critical appraisal tools available and finding the most appropriate one can be challenging. For example, Majid and Vanstone (2018) reviewed the appraisal tools available and identified over a hundred! In 2012, Hannes and Macaitis identified 24 different assessment tools that were commonly used in studies. They also found the ability of these critical appraisal tools to help identify the methodological weaknesses of the research reviewed to be variable at best. In the early 2000s, Katrak et al. (2004) also identified more than a hundred critical appraisal tools in the literature but concluded that many of them lacked any rigorous evaluation of their effectiveness; the authors argued that the proliferation of appraisal tools had not been accompanied by a thorough assessment of their value. In view of the many appraisal tools available, you will likely find a tool that is directly related to the specific type of study you need to appraise; however, it is important to remember that this tool might not have been thoroughly tested and should be regarded as an aid to encourage you to think critically about the study.

Some papers have compared the critical evaluation of studies by researchers both with and without the use of an appraisal tool. For example, Dixon-Woods et al. (2007) compared the use of two checklists and the unprompted judgement of the reader in the conclusions made about a qualitative paper. The readers were experienced researchers. They did not find that structured appraisal tools yielded more agreement about the quality of the study than unprompted judgement, although those using structured tools were more explicit in their reasons for their judgements.

The consensus is that critical appraisal tools are not an essential component of the process of critical appraisal and there is no one 'gold standard', although they are recommended for post-graduate students. Burls believed that checklists are useful not as a replacement for thought and judgement but as an 'aide memoire' (2009: 3) when considering the strengths and weaknesses of a study design. If you do decide to use a critical appraisal tool, remember you still need to possess a thorough knowledge and understanding of the research or other evidence you are evaluating.

Can artificial intelligence help with critical appraisal?

At the time of writing, there are many AI platforms that can provide a summary of a piece of research. They might even provide a critical summary. We do not consider that these are a substitute for undertaking a full critical appraisal for two reasons. First, it is important that you understand the research that you are reading and can identify the strengths and weaknesses of each study. Second, AI might not identify the strengths and weaknesses as appropriate for your study, as the nuances of searching require judgement not currently available with AI tools. However, do check your appraisal with an AI summary to determine whether it might augment your own analysis and judgement.

Examples of critical appraisal tools for empirical research

Due to the widespread availability and choice of critical appraisal tools, there are many ways to access them. One of the most useful websites is that provided by the University of South Australia, which provides links to a wide variety of critical appraisal tools for research and other sources of evidence (at time of writing this is available at: https://guides.library.unisa.edu.au/SystematicReviews/CriticalAppraisal).

Some critical appraisal tools are specific to individual research designs, for example the Critical Appraisal Skills Programme (CASP) guidelines and those published by the Joanna Briggs Institute, which publishes critical appraisal checklists for a range of studies (qualitative studies are included in one checklist). These checklists are available online at: www.casp-uk.net and https://jbi.global/critical-appraisal-tools.

Other critical appraisal tools are more general, refer to qualitative or quantitative research designs (rather than individual research designs), and are referenced in journal articles or textbooks (e.g. Law et al. 1998; Walsh and Downe 2006; Coughlan et al. 2007; Ryan et al. 2007;

Beck 2009). A critical appraisal tool for mixed-methods studies has been developed by Hawker et al. (2002), in which they recommend researchers grade the following aspects of a study from 'good' to 'very poor' and comment on why they did so:

- Abstract and title
- Introduction and aims
- Method and data
- Sampling
- Ethics and bias
- Findings/results
- Transferability and generalizability
- Implications and usefulness.

Other critical appraisal tools can be found by a simple Google search or perhaps referred to in other research textbooks and journal articles. Some critical appraisal tools provide a method of scoring a study while others provide a checklist but without a final score. Whichever type of appraisal tool you use, the important thing is that you use it to determine the strength of evidence that a paper provides for your study.

Anyone undertaking a systematic review with a meta-analysis needs to decide on the use of scales and checklists for assessing quality. While the use of numerical scores is appealing, as a method it is not supported by empirical evidence (Emerson et al. 1990; Schulz et al. 1995). Calculating a summary score inevitably involves assigning 'weights' to different items in the scale, and it is difficult to justify the weights assigned. Higgins et al. (2024) argue that it is preferable to use simple approaches for assessing validity that can be fully reported. The Cochrane Collaboration has developed a risk of bias assessment tool for use within a systematic review that incorporates RCTs (Higgins et al. 2024). This assessment tool focuses on the assessment of the risk of bias in the following areas: generation of allocation sequence, concealment of allocation, blinding, attrition, generic biases, biases specific to the trial and biases of the clinical speciality.

Examples of critical appraisal approaches for non-research evidence

In addition to critical appraisal tools for empirical research, there are also tools for assessing the quality of other evidence such as theories, guidelines, government reports, and discussion or argument papers. Such tools are now well established and are readily available; for example, the Joanna Briggs Institute has tools for the appraisal of policy and discussion (McArthur et al. 2020) on their website. Given the influence and importance that some non-research literature can have, it is important that you subject it to as much scrutiny as empirical research (Bradshaw 2015). Therefore, when you include non-research evidence in your review, it is important that you assess the quality of it in an appropriate way. For example, Dunleavy (2015, via email) undertook a systematic review to explore the barriers and facilitators to patient and carer recruitment to RCTs in palliative care. The data for this study came not only from the results of trials but also from the discussion sections, where the researchers published their reflections on the process of recruitment. Some discussions will be stronger and more logical than others and this can be assessed within a critical framework. Examples of appraisal tools for non-research evidence are given below.

Fawcett (2005) proposes criteria for the evaluation of theories and suggests that they can be considered according to:

- Significance
- Internal consistency
- Clarity
- Testability
- Confirmability with empirical research.

Bradshaw (2015) has provided a framework against which government reports can be evaluated and suggests the following criteria, which are based on the framework proposed in Thiselton (2012):

- The value judgements made by the writer of the report
- The accessibility of the report to a lay reader
- Consideration of the perceptions of the reader
- The intention to change perceptions
- The reliability of data used in the report
- Consideration of historical underpinnings
- The intention of the report.

The AGREE Collaboration (at time of writing, available at: https://www.agreetrust.org/wp-content/uploads/2013/10/AGREE-II-Users-Manual-and-23-item-Instrument_2009_UPDATE_2013.pdf) provides assessment criteria for the evaluation of clinical guidelines. The development and work of the organization is described by Brouwers et al. (2010). The aim of the criteria is to assess the methodological rigour and transparency with which the guidelines have been developed. The criteria have six domains:

- Scope and purpose
- Stakeholder involvement
- Rigour of development
- Clarity
- Applicability
- Editorial independence.

Cottrell (2011) proposes criteria for the evaluation of arguments and discusses how the author's position, line of reasoning and intention to persuade can be used to assess the quality of their argument. This approach builds on the work of Thouless and Thouless (1953), who articulate 38 'dishonest tricks' commonly used in argument, such as:

- Using emotionally charged words
- Making statements using words such as 'all' when 'some' would be more appropriate
- Using selected instances
- Misrepresentation of opposing arguments
- Evasion of a sound refutation of an argument.

How to use the critical appraisal within your literature review

The process of critical appraisal and the use of critical appraisal tools are well established within academic institutions, and many students commencing post-graduate study will be familiar with them. It can be tempting to see critical appraisal as an 'end in itself' rather than a method that will assist your ongoing analysis and synthesis of literature. When you undertake your critical appraisal, it is important that you make judgement as to the overall strengths and weaknesses of the research or other evidence that you have, as you will base your subsequent analysis and synthesis on these.

In summary

Critical appraisal enables you to identify the strengths and weaknesses of a paper and hence determine the weight given to that paper in your subsequent analysis. We argue that an appropriate critical appraisal tool can be a useful way of considering quality issues in a research paper.

However, it is important to remember that the process of critical appraisal is not synonymous with the use of a tool. The use of a tool should prompt you to think critically about the research or other evidence you are using for your review. You can also think critically about the literature without the use of a tool. Use of a critical appraisal tool is not a substitute for a sound knowledge of the research methods used in a paper, without which it is not possible to appraise it. There are many critical appraisal tools available; you may find it helpful to use a tool that is specific to the research design you are using rather than a generic tool. In recent years, the Cochrane Collaboration has moved away from the use of traditional critical appraisal tools towards tools that focus explicitly on the risk of bias. Anyone undertaking a systematic review with meta-analysis is advised to refer to the risk of bias assessment tool in Higgins et al. (2024). Once you have made a critical appraisal of a study, and have identified its strengths and weaknesses, you need to decide how you will use that appraisal in your literature review. We will discuss this in Chapter 7.

Key points

- Critical appraisal enables you to determine the strengths and weaknesses of the papers in your review
- Critical appraisal or risk of bias tools can be a useful aid to this processIt is possible to appraise a paper without the use of a tool
- A critical appraisal does is not a substitute for understanding the methods used in a paper
- Critical appraisal is not a 'standalone' activity
- Critical appraisal should be used within your subsequent data analysis and synthesis.

7

How do I analyse and synthesize my literature?

In this chapter, we will discuss:

- *The different approaches to the analysis and synthesis of literature*
- *How the approach to analysis and synthesis depends on the method you undertake for your review*
- *Give some examples of types of synthesis methods*
- *Describe elements common to all synthesis.*

You will have now selected the research and other evidence that is relevant for your literature review. This will comprise the research papers and other evidence that meet your inclusion criteria, which may have stated methodological requirements for inclusion in the review. You will have undertaken a data extraction and a critical appraisal of all included studies. You will now have a working knowledge of which are the stronger and which are the weaker papers in your review. You are now ready to analyse and synthesize your literature:

- *Analysis*: breaking down the parts in order to understand the individual components
- *Synthesis*: building up the parts into a coherent whole.

Data extraction and critical appraisal will form the first stage of your analysis. You will continue your analysis when you look closely at the details of what each paper can tell you about your review question. In your synthesis, you will build a picture of what all the papers can tell you about your review question.

Different methods of analysis and synthesis are required for different types of data – that is, whether you have quantitative or qualitative research, or a mixture of both and/or other evidence. You should be familiar with the data analysis used in quantitative and qualitative research. In quantitative research, data is often analysed and synthesized numerically, using statistical tests, with a critique, whereas in qualitative research, texts are analysed and synthesized without numbers. The same approaches are applied to the analysis and synthesis of literature in a review.

Quantitative papers that are sufficiently similar can be analysed and synthesized using statistical analysis known as a meta-analysis or descriptive statistics. The methods have been developed over many years and there are high levels of agreement about the approach. Qualitative papers can be analysed and synthesized thematically and there are many approaches to doing so. As mentioned in Chapter 2, there is methodological debate about the appropriateness of combining different qualitative approaches (Atkins et al. 2008), but there is general agreement that the utility of bringing evidence together in an analysis and synthesis outweighs methodological considerations such as loss of context, if the review is undertaken rigorously.

Going beyond describing the content of original studies is often referred to as the defining characteristic of analysis and synthesis (Harden et al. 2004). It is the main purpose of a literature review to bring all the results of the studies together in an appropriate analysis and synthesis. The way in which you undertake this analysis and synthesis of your literature depends on the type of literature that you have and the approach to the literature review that you have undertaken.

In this chapter, we will discuss the analysis of literature using statistical measures and non-statistical approaches. In Chapter 2, we listed some of the different approaches to doing a literature review (see Table 2.1). We are going to use these classifications in this chapter to give an overview of the methods of synthesis and suggest when each might be applicable.

Systematic reviews with meta-analysis

Meta-analysis may be appropriate for your review if the papers you have selected for analysis are quantitative, often randomized controlled trials, and adopt a similar method and have similar outcomes.

Meta-analysis is a statistical re-analysis of the original data in the individual papers to provide one overall statistical result.

In the same way that the Cochrane approach to systematic review was the forerunner of the literature review as a formal research method, meta-analysis was one of the first formal and standardized approaches to data analysis. Meta-analysis has been crucial to the development of evidence-based practice. In the example given in Chapter 1, the effectiveness of streptokinase, a drug used in the treatment of myocardial infarction, was identified through a meta-analysis of many small clinical trials (Mulrow 1994). Due to the small sample size of each individual trial, most could not find conclusively in favour of the use of streptokinase. However, when the trials were brought together in a meta-analysis, and the samples and results were pooled and re-analysed, the true effect of the drug became apparent.

Meta-analysis is a means of combining findings from similar studies to arrive at an overall outcome, based on a summary of the results of all those studies. This means that effect sizes of individual studies can be combined to form a summary statistic to show the effect size across studies. Typical effect sizes used include risk ratio, relative risk and odds ratio. This procedure is only possible when studies include outcome data recorded in such a way that you can identify or calculate the effect size and when the studies all used the same outcome measures. This is most likely to be the case in intervention studies. Meta-analysis usually includes RCTs or quasi-RCTs because these studies provide the best evidence to base decisions on. The results of the studies can be combined statistically. However, many RCTs are also at high risk of bias, highlighting that no research is perfect and we should always be aware of the limitations involved. You can run a meta-analysis with all studies included and then run it again without the poorer-quality ones to determine whether there is any real difference in omitting the latter.

A meta-analysis is often the end point of a systematic review and is often presented visually in a diagram referred to as a forest plot. Clear instructions on undertaking a meta-analysis can be found in the *Cochrane Handbook for Systematic Reviews of Interventions* (Higgins et al. 2024). This is an online handbook that is divided into chapters that are searchable, which makes it easier to use.

The forest plot (diagram of a meta-analysis) shown in Figure 7.2 is taken from a systematic review in which the authors reviewed studies of changes in the mental health outcomes (e.g. anxiety, mixed anxiety and depression, depression and stress) both of people who had stopped smoking and those who continued to smoke (Taylor et al. 2014). The aim of the study was to investigate the commonly held belief that increased stress and mental health problems are a barrier to smoking cessation. The authors pooled the results of 26 longitudinal studies that had assessed the mental health of participants who had continued to smoke and participants who had stopped smoking. They found that the participants who had stopped smoking experienced a significantly improved quality of life compared with those who continued to smoke, providing evidence that smoking cessation does not lead to additional stress, as is often claimed.

As well as providing a summary statistic – related to the improvement in mental health of the participants who had quit smoking – you could perform a sensitivity analysis to determine the impact of a particular study based, for example, on study quality. Or you could conduct a sub-group analysis to see if a particular population characteristic impacts your findings. You will still need to describe your findings and offer a critique of the included studies. This might include a critique of the study design which may have resulted in differing findings.

Presentation of a forest plot

In Figure 7.1, all of the individual studies are listed on the left-hand side of the plot. The measured difference in the mean mental health score between the participants who stopped smoking and the participants who did not is represented by the small square in the middle of each horizontal line. If the data are binary (i.e. a system that uses only two values: 0 and 1), this is often presented as an odds ratio or risk ratio but in this study the data are continuous. The horizontal line represents the confidence intervals for the study. The confidence intervals can be taken to represent the uncertainty about the effect of stopping smoking on change in mental health. Confidence intervals are explained below.

A line of 'no effect' runs down the middle of the chart. Any study where the confidence intervals cross this line indicates there is no evidence of a difference between the mental health of those who stopped smoking and those who did not, so it is a non-significant result. In this forest plot, you can see that many of the studies show benefits in the mental health of the participants who stopped smoking.

The weight of each study is presented as a percentage, which reflects how strongly each study contributes to the overall average effect estimate. More precise studies, those with narrower confidence intervals, contribute more weight to the overall average.

The diamond represents the average of all studies' results. The vertical points of the diamond lie on the average of all studies, and the

Study	SE	Weight (%)	Standard mean difference (95% CI)
Anxiety			
Solomon 2006	0.19	25	−0.06 (−0.42 to 0.30)
Dawkins 2009	0.25	20	−0.19 (−0.68 to 0.30)
McDermott 2013	0.13	29	−0.74 (−1.00 to −0.48)
Becona 2002	0.18	26	−0.37 (−0.72 to −0.02)
Total		100	−0.37 (−0.70 to −0.03)
Test for heterogeneity: τ^2=0.08, χ^2=10.43, df=3, P=0.02, I^2=71%			
Test for overall effect: z=2.16, P=0.03			
Depression			
Solomon 2006	0.19	9	0.01 (−0.35 to 0.37)
Berlin 2010	0.22	7	−0.30 (−0.72 to 0.12)
Blalock 2008	0.22	7	−0.58 (−1.00 to −0.16)
Dawkins 2009	0.25	5	−0.39 (−0.88 to 0.10)
Kahler 2011	0.21	7	−0.28 (−0.69 to 0.13)
Vazquez 1999	0.17	11	−0.12 (−0.44 to 0.20)
Busch 2011	0.19	9	−0.30 (−0.67 to 0.07)
Kahler 2002	0.20	8	−0.69 (−1.09 to −0.29)
Munafo 2008	0.09	21	−0.09 (−0.27 to 0.09)
Kinnunen 2006	0.11	17	−0.21 (−0.42 to 0.00)
Total		100	−0.25 (−0.37 to −0.12)
Test for heterogeneity: τ^2=0.01, χ^2=12.83, df=9, P=0.17, I^2=30%			
Test for overall effect: z=3.89, P<0.001			
Mixed anxiety and depression			
Blalock 2008	0.44	4	−0.21 (−1.07 to 0.65)
Kahler 2009	0.29	8	−0.64 (−1.22 to −0.06)
Steinberg 2011	0.14	35	−0.29 (−0.57 to −0.01)
Mino 2000	0.26	10	−0.44 (−0.95 to 0.07)
Chassin 2002	0.13	42	−0.23 (−0.48 to 0.02)
Total		100	−0.31 (−0.47 to −0.14)
Test for heterogeneity: τ^2=0.00, χ^2=1.94, df=4, P=0.75, I^2=0%			
Test for overall effect: z=3.61, P<0.001			
Stress			
Manning 2005	0.17	17	−0.25 (−0.58 to −0.08)
Hajek 2010	0.09	55	−0.22 (−0.40 to −0.04)
Chassin 2002	0.13	29	−0.36 (−0.61 to −0.11)
Total		100	−0.27 (−0.40 to −0.13)
Test for heterogeneity: τ^2=0.00, χ^2=0.77, df=2, P=0.68, I^2=0%			
Test for overall effect: z=3.80, P<0.001			

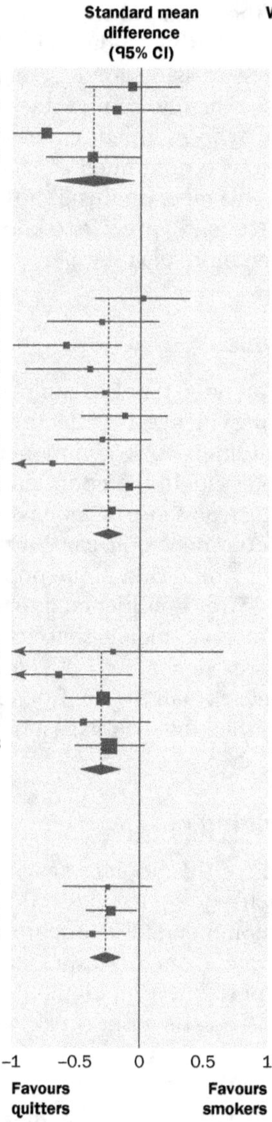

Figure 7.1 Forest plot to illustrate the changes in mental health of participants who stopped smoking and participants who did not, from the start of the study to follow-up

Source: Taylor et al. (2014)

horizontal points of the diamond represent the 95 per cent confidence interval of the average. In this study, the authors analysed each type of outcome separately (depression, anxiety and so on) and in each case the diamonds do not cross the line of no effect. Hence we can be confident that the participants who stopped smoking had better mental health than the participants who continued to smoke and that this cannot be put down to chance. This meta-analysis shows that each individual study was generally not sufficiently precise to know this, but the average of all of them gives us much more certainty.

Confidence intervals

The confidence we can have that the sample is an accurate indication of the true population prevalence is reflected in the confidence intervals, which give numerical limits to a 'common-sense' approach. Confidence intervals are used to estimate the confidence that the sample reflects a range within which the true score is known to lie. The smaller the interval or range, the more confident you can be that the results of the study reflect the results you would find in the population at large. Using a formula, the upper and lower confidence intervals can be calculated. A 95 per cent confidence interval means that we can be 95 per cent sure that the true population prevalence lies between the lower and upper confidence interval. However small the confidence intervals are, if they cross the line of 'no effect', then this confirms a non-significant result.

Meta-analysis training

It is beyond the scope of this book to describe the process of meta-analysis in detail. If you are going to undertake meta-analysis, then further training would be recommended. There are various courses available or you could seek advice from a statistician or experienced reviewer. If you are going to perform a meta-analysis, then consider whether it would be suitable to register your work as a Cochrane review. Some PhD students have successfully done this but you do need to be working with a team of researchers. Initially, you attempt to register your title with a specific group in Cochrane and if they want to pursue this, you are given access to their editors and to their software, RevMan. RevMan is a database designed to run and report on systematic reviews. The first step is to write a protocol for the systematic review you intend to undertake, describing the methods for the main review. You would need to discuss this in detail with your supervisor.

Analysis when a meta-analysis is not possible

As discussed in Chapter 2, it is not always possible to conduct a meta-analysis. Many systematic reviews do not involve a meta-analysis. There are many reasons for this, including insufficient detail in the data or a series of studies that are very different from one another. This is sometimes referred to as heterogeneous data. You may also find that the only data available relate to other types of quantitative papers – such as a case series with a before-and-after design – and not RCTs. It would still be possible to use the data from such studies in descriptive form, sometimes referred to as a narrative analysis, rather than to create a summary statistic, or meta-analysis. For those of you undertaking a narrative analysis, you would need to describe who took part in the study and say if all participants were included in the analysis. You would describe the different effect sizes, whether results were all in favour of a treatment or not, and any discrepancies in results. It is important to identify the limitations of the findings and the likelihood that the results will lead to the need for a definitive study in the future.

If you include research which is considered to be less rigorous, for example a case series, it is important to remember that these studies are at a higher risk of bias because they have not been designed to include blinding, randomization or other forms of comparison (although sometimes participants are compared before and after the measure). Therefore, it is not possible to rule out the impact of other variables upon the outcome of the study. For example, deterioration in disease state can confound the results of before-and-after studies, which would be controlled for in an RCT.

In addition to the use of descriptive statistics to describe your findings, you will also need to provide a narrative summary of what you found. The approach to narrative synthesis described by Popay et al. (2006) is an example of this. Popay et al. (2006) define the process of a narrative synthesis (below), emphasizing the thematic and content analysis of the data, which has clear parallels with the analysis of qualitative and mixed-methods research.

- Identification of theory (optional)
- Textual description of the data
- Tabulation of the data
- Thematic and content analysis of the data
- Reciprocal translation (similarities in the data)
- Refutational translation (differences in the data).

As mentioned in Chapter 2, there are reporting guidelines to help develop your understanding of conducting your review without a meta-analysis. This is called Synthesis Without Meta-Analysis (SWiM) in systematic reviews (Campbell et al. 2020).

> **Example**
> An example of a systematic review without meta-analysis using the SWiM guidelines is that of Jurd and Barr (2024). They wished to explore the role of leadership factors and their impact on cardiopulmonary resuscitation. They were unable to complete a meta-analysis and instead followed the SWiM guidelines. Quite a few papers using SWiM do not include a synthesis method but that of Jurd and Barr does. Rather than following Popay, they adopted a qualitive analysis method more commonly used to analyse interview data (Braun and Clarke 2006).

Descriptive mapping reviews

As we have described above, a statistical approach to the analysis and synthesis of data is often not appropriate, even when the data are numerical in nature. There are many alternative approaches to data analysis when doing a literature review. Descriptive mapping reviews, our next category, present the data in a logical, categorial manner and do not attempt further interpretation. These approaches to the analysis of literature are influenced by the logic of the Cochrane approach to systematic reviews with meta-analysis, many of which have been developed to provide an approach to analysis when meta-analysis is out of the question.

Meta-aggregation

Meta-aggregation, for example, developed by researchers at the Joanna Briggs Institute, is a pragmatic strategy for analysing mainly qualitative and other data that do not lend themselves to a meta-analysis. The approach is described as aggregative, or putting together, and does not explicitly encourage a re-interpretation of the literature in the review.

However, the complexity of interpretative and critical understanding of the complex phenomena involved in qualitative research is acknowledged. The aim of a meta-aggregation is the product of pragmatic and generalizable statements, together with recommendations for practice with an emphasis on guidance for action.

The focus of data analysis is inductive rather than the predominantly deductive approach of a framework analysis. Hannes and Lockwood (2011) identify the following process:

- The findings of studies are assembled into themes, categories and metaphors
- Phase 1 themes are identified by the original research papers
- Phase 2 themes are identified through further analysis
- Common themes across all papers are identified
- Declamatory statements or lines of action are identified.

Hannes and Lockwood emphasize the importance of keeping to the original data in the literature analysis and synthesis, and refer to the method of constant comparison analysis as described by Lincoln and Guba (1985). Despite the reference to interpretation in a meta-aggregation, Hannes and Lockwood (2011) emphasize that a meta-aggregation works best for the synthesis of findings where the concepts are clearly defined and well specified and where there is a clear relationship between the themes identified in the individual research paper and the final declamatory statements or lines of action. The emphasis of meta-aggregation is on the development of pragmatic lines of action that move beyond the generation of theory and can form recommendations for practice.

Example

A meta-aggregation was undertaken by Jakimowicz et al. (2015) into patients' subjective experience of nurse-led clinics. The researchers undertook a comprehensive search, according to pre-defined inclusion and exclusion criteria. They identified 11 papers that met their criteria. Critical appraisal was undertaken but all of the studies were included. Significant findings were identified and aggregated into categories. Sets of statements representing the categories were produced.

Scoping review

A scoping review is another descriptive means of presenting data. As discussed in Chapter 2, it lacks the depth of other review methods but allows for an area to be mapped out and described, which helps inform us of what research has already been conducted. In particular, it may highlight the current state of knowledge in an under-researched area. There is no formal synthesis, rather studies are described and grouped. The outline for a scoping review is as follows:

Stage 1: Identifying the research question
Stage 2: Identifying relevant studies
Stage 3: Study selection
Stage 4: Charting the data
Stage 5: Collating, summarizing and reporting the results.

Example
Dodd et al. (2020) conducted a scoping review on 'Understanding the outcomes of supplementary support services in palliative care for older people'. They wanted to understand these outcomes from a stakeholder perspective so they could map them against known outcome tool measurements. This is an under-researched and rather niche area so there was little research on the topic. The authors also wanted to use the review findings to help them select outcome measures for a future research project. They noted the usefulness of a scoping review to help explore the area. They used the method of Arksey and O'Malley (2005) with enhancements by Levac et al. (2010) which help clarify and define the key stages of Arksey and O'Malley's method. As is usual in a scoping review, no quality assessments were made.

Qualitative evidence synthesis

If all of your literature is qualitative, you might consider a qualitative evidence synthesis. Of the various options available to you, many are derived from established approaches to the analysis of qualitative data and are similar in the methods they use. We will first explore one of the more established methods: meta-ethnography.

Meta-ethnography

This was one of the first methods to address the process of literature analysis and synthesis. It was described by Noblit and Hare (1988) in what has become one of the most referred-to works in the field. Although the approach was written initially for the analysis and synthesis of ethnographic studies, the authors state that it can be used with all types of qualitative research, and there are many examples of this in the literature (Campbell et al. 2011; Toye et al. 2014). The hallmark of meta-ethnography is its focus on interpretation rather than aggregation or data summary. The approach was developed in order to avoid what the authors refer to as context stripping, the incomplete and simplistic analysis and synthesis of qualitative evidence. Instead, Noblit and Hare (1988) sought an alternative approach to the analysis and synthesis of qualitative research that captured the essence and depth of the qualitative studies to be included in a review without being too 'reductionist' – or over-simplifying complex data into neatly packaged outcomes.

In combining the studies, Noblit and Hare sought to identify the complexity of the relationships between the themes in the various studies, the aim of which is 'to make the obvious obvious, the obvious dubious or the hidden obvious' (Noblit and Hare 1988: 17).

The interpretation of literature included in a meta-ethnography is the product of the analysis and synthesis of all of the papers included in the review. The results of the review are interpretative and explanatory rather than 'concrete' (Noblit and Hare 1988: 32).

Noblit and Hare (1988) refer to the work of Lincoln and Guba (1985), who describe the process of constant comparative analysis, a technique for the analysis of qualitative data that is based on the work of Glaser and Strauss (1967). Noblit and Hare applied the established process of constant comparative analysis of qualitative data (raw data collected for the purposes of a qualitative research study) to the analysis and synthesis of completed qualitative research studies, so allowing one study to be compared against another.

This constant comparative approach is described as the basis of data analysis and synthesis in a meta-ethnography and its aim is 'a new, integrated, and more complete interpretation of findings that offers greater understanding in depth and breadth than findings from individual studies' (Bondas and Hall 2007: 115).

The aim of the constant comparative approach to the analysis and synthesis of qualitative research is to achieve greater interpretative and explanatory power than a more aggregative or summative approach would allow. This process is 'one that involves opening up spaces for new insights and understandings to emerge rather than one in which totalising concepts are valued over richness and thickness of description' (Walsh and Downe 2005: 205).

As discussed in Chapter 2, meta-ethnography is an approach to undertaking a literature review where the reviewer does not always conduct a comprehensive search of the literature, although many do. Noblit and Hare (1988) argue that it might not be necessary to locate every study and that the conceptual synthesis will not be affected if five rather than ten studies are located, if they contain the same concept. The assumption is that the ten studies will contain the same concepts as five, and that the unidentified literature will not shed new light on the literature review question. This entails a judgement to be made that would need to be defended in the reviewer's written work or oral examination. The decision whether or not to conduct a comprehensive search will have an effect on the subsequent data analysis. Data analysis in a meta-ethnography involves comparing the results of the different studies included in the review. In order to do this, the results sections of the research papers are 'coded', which we describe later in this chapter, so that key concepts are identified from each study and then compared to determine whether they can be identified in other studies. Noblit and Hare (1988) refer to this process as 'translating concepts into one another'. In other words, the studies are closely compared with one another. In this method, the themes identified in the results of one research paper are compared with themes that are similar in another research paper. This is referred to as reciprocal translation. Themes that illustrate opposing ideas and concepts are also compared with each other. This is referred to as refutational translation, or the analysis of deviant themes. The end result of the synthesis is the development of a line of argument, which is similar to, but less practically orientated than, the lines of action developed by someone undertaking a meta-aggregation.

Analysis of literature in a meta-ethnography involves:

- Identifying a research question
- Reading the studies
- Identifying how the studies are related
- Translating the studies into one another
- Considering reciprocal (similar) aspects of the data
- Considering refutational (deviant) aspects of the data
- Synthesizing, or developing a line of argument.

In Noblit and Hare's initial description of meta-ethnography (1988), they do not mention critical appraisal of the included studies, although they acknowledge that all studies, irrespective of quality, will be included in the review. The argument for omitting a quality assessment is that although studies of poorer quality will add less to the understanding of the literature as a whole, they will not 'distort' the analysis. Subsequent advances in the analysis and synthesis of qualitative research have developed the role of critical appraisal, which we will discuss later in this chapter.

Example

Toye et al. (2014) used a meta-ethnographic approach to investigate female patients' experiences of chronic pelvic pain. In their review, they did strive for a comprehensive approach to literature searching, acknowledging that this approach is not always promoted in a meta-ethnography review. They undertook a quality appraisal but did not exclude studies on the basis of quality. Key concepts were then identified and compared across the studies using a constant comparative analysis in order to construct a line of argument about the experience of chronic pain and the effect it has on women's lives.

Since the publication of Noblit and Hare's (1988) seminal work, various adaptations of meta-ethnography have been developed. One reason for this is the association of meta-ethnography with ethnographic studies. Although Noblit and Hare (1988) state that their approach can be applied to qualitative studies other than ethnography, there is an obvious assumption that, because of its name, meta-ethnography is exclusively a method for the analysis and synthesis of ethnographic studies. Consequently, many approaches to qualitative research synthesis and analysis have been developed from

Noblit and Hare's original work that emphasize the importance of comprehensive searching, critical appraisal, analysis and synthesis of a wide range of qualitative and mixed-methods approaches.

Thematic synthesis

Developed by Thomas and Harden (2008), this is another approach that is closely related to meta-ethnography but which incorporates the analysis of all types of qualitative research. Thomas and Harden (2008) developed their approach from a series of studies investigating barriers to and facilitators of mental health, healthy eating and physical activity in young people (Thomas et al. 2003; Harden et al. 2004) and pregnancy support for young people (Harden et al. 2006).

In their approach, Harden et al. (2006) refer to the 'aggregation' of studies, although in this context it is apparent that they are referring to the interpretation rather than 'pooling' of qualitative studies. This illustrates that terms such as 'aggregation' can be used differently in different contexts and it is important to understand the meaning behind the descriptions of the methods used.

Harden and his colleagues' (2006) description of a thematic analysis is another example of an approach to undertaking a literature review where the reviewers do not conduct a comprehensive search of the literature but instead use a sample of relevant literature.

Thomas and Harden's (2008) approach to thematic synthesis involves the following steps:

- Identifying a research question
- Purposive searching, aiming for conceptual saturation rather than a comprehensive inclusion of all literature
- Quality appraisal, recognizing the complexity of this process
- Identifying key concepts in individual studies
- Developing codes and themes from the key concepts
- Checking of consistency of coding/themes between the different studies
- 'Translating concepts into one another'
- Generating themes; third-order interpretations.

Thomas and Harden describe in detail how they coded and began to develop themes, coding each line of text according to its meaning and content (2008: 3). They describe the translation of one concept into another as a key task of qualitative research synthesis, referring to the work of Britten et al. (2002) and Noblit and Hare (1988). If you compare the methods described by Noblit and Hare (1988) and Thomas and Harden (2008), it can be argued that third-order interpretations as described by Thomas and Harden (2008) are equivalent to third-order interpretations of meta-ethnography (Noblit and Hare 1988), and that the reviewers infer from the descriptive themes in order to address the question posed by the literature review. Thus the two approaches have many similarities with some differences in the method regarding searching and critical appraisal.

For example, in their systematic review of the barriers to and facilitators of healthy eating, Thomas and Harden (2008) found a common theme in many individual studies, in that children are attracted by 'tasty' rather than 'healthy' food. In their synthesis, they were able to infer that it would be beneficial to brand fruit as 'tasty' rather than 'healthy'. They refer to this synthesis as a third-order interpretation.

Example

Thematic synthesis was the approach used by a qualitative systematic review published by the Cochrane Collaboration (Glenton et al. 2013), widely cited as being the first systematic review of qualitative research. In this review, researchers investigated the barriers to and facilitators of the implementation of lay health workers in an attempt to improve access to maternal child health. Glenton et al. used a purposive sample of research in their review, as advocated by Thomas and Harden (2008), rather than a fully comprehensive search. A critical appraisal was undertaken and all studies were included in the review. The researchers used an *a priori* framework approach for the analysis of data, adding new themes where these were indicated by a study. The results were charted and the similarities and differences between the individual studies were summarized. The concepts were then defined and interpreted. The researchers described the data in the studies as providing a 'thin' rather than a 'thick' description of the concepts, although their conclusions portray a comprehensive description and understanding of the role of a lay healthcare worker, including the motivation for the role and how there can be tensions between those providing lay and professional care services.

Meta-synthesis

This is another approach to the analysis and synthesis of qualitative research. The term was first defined shortly before the introduction of meta-ethnography by Stern and Harris in 1985 and is described by Walsh and Downe (2005). Like thematic synthesis, this approach is closely related to meta-ethnography and also incorporates the principles of constant comparative analysis as described by Lincoln and Guba (1985) and Glaser and Strauss (1967). Similar to a meta-ethnography and thematic synthesis, the aims of meta-synthesis are the interpretation of qualitative research findings in order to gain new insight from a body of literature that would not be apparent from the studies viewed in isolation. Thorne et al. (2004: 1358) describe the aim of meta-synthesis as providing

> *integrations that are more than the sum of the parts, in that they offer novel interpretations of findings. These interpretations will not be found in any one research report but rather are inferences derived from taking all of the reports in a sample as a whole.*

The key features of a meta-analysis approach are described by Walsh and Downe (2005). Significantly, unlike meta-ethnography and thematic synthesis, Walsh and Downe (2005) recommend a comprehensive rather than a selective or purposive search strategy. As Barroso et al. recommend, 'for researchers conducting qualitative meta-synthesis projects, the ideal goal is to retrieve all of the relevant studies in a field, not just a sample of them' (2003: 153).

Walsh and Downe (2005) recommend that a critical appraisal of the literature is undertaken but acknowledge that this is a contested area and one that might not be easily resolved, especially with qualitative research papers, about which it can be difficult to achieve agreement as to what constitutes quality. The steps described by Walsh and Downe (2005) are:

- Comprehensive search for relevant studies
- Reading and re-reading of the studies
- Critical appraisal of the studies
- Description of how the studies are related
- Analysis, in which key metaphors are compared and contrasted
- Identification of themes
- Organization of themes into a table/grid of key content
- Translation of studies into each other
- Identification of themes as reciprocal (similar) or refutational (contrasting)
- Avoidance of 'force fitting'
- Preservation of the original text to retain richness
- Synthesis of translation: more refined meanings.

Integrative and mixed-methods reviews

Integrative and mixed-methods reviews incorporate research from different paradigms. The method of analysis for these types of literature review thus needs to reflect this diversity, and often reflects the way in which qualitative data is analysed, so you might use methods as outlined in the section above. From discussion of the methods of analysis in meta-ethnography, thematic synthesis and meta-synthesis, you can see the subtle differences in the methods for data analysis within the range of literature reviews available. This is not without debate (Jensen and Allen 1996; Rogers et al. 1996). Atkins et al. (2008) even question whether different types of qualitative research can be combined in one study, given the different philosophical positions from which they emerged. Although this might seem logical, it does not take into account the fact that many different forms of evidence might be relevant to an individual review question and that the utility of combining studies in a review might outweigh the conceptual arguments against doing so. Further developments have seen approaches that advocate the combining of different types of research and other evidence. Harden and Thomas (2005) argue that research questions should not be confined in their answers by the type of study but by relevance of the study to the research question and hence incorporate a range of studies in their reviews. Harden and Thomas recommend that the results of a diverse range of evidence can be analysed using a systematic approach. Although we include thematic synthesis under qualitative evidence synthesis methods, it is a versatile method that can also be used to incorporate data from different types of studies.

Given this debate, you are advised to adhere closely to the method of analysis proposed and described in your chosen method and have a clear rationale for doing so. The principle to consider is that the method of analysis should reflect the paradigm in which the research is situated (Booth 2019); that is, the analysis of qualitative and quantitative papers should consider the depth of data within the papers and should not be reduced to a series of lists (Thorne 2017), as to do so would reduce a rich data set to a single concept and risk mis-representing the data. For example, Whittemore and Knafl (2005) suggest using the constant comparative method – the method used to analyse data in grounded theory – as a method for data analysis in an integrative review. Data are compared item by item so that similar data can be compared and grouped together in order to identify themes, patterns and relationships. Data can be displayed as a matrix or table. The key elements of their review method are as follows:

- Problem identification
- Literature search
- Data evaluation
- Data analysis
- Conclusion
- Verification

Examples

Walsh et al. (2024) used Whittemore and Knafl's (2005) method in their integrated literature review which explored 'Preregistration nursing students' motivation for speaking up for patient safety'. They used the JBI critical appraisal tool to determine the quality of the studies, a tool that can be used for any methodological design. Of the 27 studies included in their review, 18 were quantitative, one was mixed methods and six used a range of qualitative designs. Interestingly, the authors also included an integrative review and a concept analysis, which is unusual in an integrative review.

In another example, in their study of care and support needs of people who look after adults at risk of suicide, Lascelles et al. (2024) undertook a mixed-methods review employing Thomas and Harden's (2008) approach to thematic synthesis. The authors had a mix of qualitative and quantitative papers and undertook data transformation to combine the qualitative with the quantitative research. Descriptive themes were first developed followed by analytical themes.

Paradigm or theory-driven approaches

Paradigm or theory-driven reviews focus on the development of theory rather than the aggregation or integration of data as an end in itself. Data analysis can be approached in various ways, including using the methods discussed in previous sections of this book. Take, for example, critical interpretive synthesis, a method discussed in Chapter 2. Dixon-Woods et al. (2006) emphasize the need to undertake interpretive synthesis involving induction and interpretation in order to facilitate the development of concepts and theories. The same authors also refer to a 'line of argument' synthesis, which they describe as a 'synthesizing argument'. Specifically, critical interpretive synthesis involves looking for similarities in the data (reciprocal analysis) and differences in the data (refutational analysis) in order to produce a synthesizing argument. Dixon-Woods et al. (2006) argue that:

> *this argument integrates evidence from across the studies in the review into a coherent theoretical framework comprising a network of constructs and relationships between them. Its function is to provide more insightful, formalized and generalizable ways of understanding phenomena.*

Data analysis in a paradigm or theory-driven review seeks to incorporate acknowledgement of the paradigm in which the research is located in addition to the actual research study, and incorporates both the paradigm and the study findings in the analysis. In many approaches, research is generally compared initially from within its own paradigm so that any inconsistencies within the data can be reviewed within the paradigm in which it was described. In order to ensure that research from different research traditions can be incorporated, data analysis is often undertaken following the principles of qualitative data analysis, for example as described by Denzin and Lincoln (1994). The goal of the review is to find explanations for differences in findings and recommendations made by researchers in different traditions.

Realist review

A realist review is an example of a theory-driven review which has as its focus, understanding what works, why and how in a specific context. Realist reviews often use the results and ideas generated by systematic review and continue to analyse why the interventions might work rather than just accepting the findings at face value, without considering contextual factors. The evidence used in a realist review is diverse, as the reviewers look to identify any contextual influences, such as theories that have triggered interest in the intervention, and consider the theoretical basis as well as the empirical basis for the interventions. In view of this, approaches to analysis are also varied with many researchers referring to both deductive and inductive logic (Fothergill et al. 2025).

Example

A realist review was undertaken by Greenhalgh et al. (2007) following the publication of a Cochrane Collaboration systematic review which identified that school meal programmes significantly improved the growth and cognitive performance of disadvantaged children. The researchers were interested in understanding which aspects of the programme worked and for whom and in what circumstances. They analysed the studies included in the systematic review using realist methods. They constructed a matrix to analyse the data concerning the nature of the experiments and any theories or mechanisms identified by the researchers as possible explanations for the success or failure of the programmes. The researchers then searched for additional theories to explain the findings. Their analysis supported the focus of school feeding programmes for disadvantaged children but recommended that for some very malnourished children, the school feeding programme could focus on providing high-energy foods to compensate for food not available at home.

Overview of reviews

Sometimes there will be a plethora of research as well as a number of reviews on your topic, in which case you can bring all these together in a review of reviews as discussed in Chapter 2. In your analysis, you will treat the reviews as your primary focus of research and the findings of the reviews as your primary data. You will be interested in comparing the findings of the different reviews, not the individual papers.

There are two established methods for doing a 'review of reviews'. The first was developed by the Cochrane Collaboration, whose method focuses on combining the results of systematic reviews with meta-analysis. Details of the method of analysis are available on their website. An alternative and more versatile method is the 'umbrella review', which was developed by the Joanna Briggs Institute (JBI). This method does not focus on systematic reviews with meta-analysis but on the inclusion of different types of review, thus making the umbrella an inclusive option for those looking to undertake a review with a wider scope. Full details of this method can be found on their website.

Example

Couto et al. (2025) conducted an umbrella review using the JBI method. They wanted to explore 'Nurse and midwife interventions to protect, promote and support breastfeeding'. They included 29 reviews, most of which they described as 'systematic reviews' but six reviews only included RCTs and three were scoping reviews. You can see why the JBI method was appropriate here. They used a critical appraisal tool specifically designed for reviews called the Critical Appraisal Checklist for Systematic reviews. They did not comment on how well this worked for the different types of reviews in the study. Two reviewers extracted the data and they identified themes across the different review findings.

Common features in the analysis of reviews where a meta-analysis is not undertaken

There are many approaches to the analysis and synthesis of qualitative and quantitative research in a review, and we refer in this book to a selection only of those you might come across. Our overall recommendation is that you identify a named approach that is appropriate for your overall method and follow it closely. There are sometimes many similarities between different methods and there might even appear to be a crossover between different approaches. Rather confusingly, you might also find that terminology is also used interchangeably. With this in mind, we have presented some of the similarities between the approaches where a meta-analysis is not undertaken.

Step 1: coding your literature

The first step is to begin to code your data. This means reading and re-reading the included papers. This is the start of the process of identifying 'themes' from results of each study that you have. It is also possible to add a qualitative code to quantitative data. To start this process of coding, go directly to the results section of each paper and re-read this section. If your paper is discussion only, then go to the general discussion section of the paper.

If you have predominantly empirical research papers, then go through the main findings and consider how you might describe the findings the researchers present. You can use the terms used in the paper or you can paraphrase the findings in your own words. These descriptions will become the initial codes that you use to describe your data. If you have mainly discussion papers or other reports, you can allocate themes to the main discussion points.

Your codes are generated from the main findings or results of a paper; each research paper is likely to contain several codes which you can then combine with the codes from other papers. When you allocate codes to the results of the different papers, try to think of words that summarize the main point that is being made in that particular section. You might choose to annotate the paper using a highlighter pen to identify the themes. Go through all your papers following this method until you have assigned a code to all the appropriate results/discussion sections of the papers.

There is a variety of software that can assist you in doing this, or alternatively you can complete this analysis on hard copies of the papers. It is important to remember that computer software packages for the non-statistical analysis of literature do not do the analysis for you – they only assist you in organizing and handling the data.

Example literature review question: *What are the experiences and perceptions of patients and nurses of the bedside handover?*

Below is an extract of the results of a study by Sand-Jecklin and Sherman (2013) in which they used a mixed-methods approach to investigate patients' experience and perceptions of the bedside handover, following implementation of this approach to communication about patient care. Possible initial coding is indicated in bold.

Independent T test comparisons revealed significantly higher scores (from patients) post implementation (of bedside handover) on 2 items: 'made sure I knew who my nurse was' **(introduction of nurse/patient)** and 'include in shift report' **(involvement in care)** ... patients were invited to add narrative comments on the post implementation survey. Of the 251 comments, 102 (42%) were positive, whereas 24 (10%) indicated that nursing staff did not use bedside report, used it inconsistently or used it only to introduce the oncoming nurse ... Nurses were asked to respond narratively in a formative evaluation of bedside report, one month post implementation. The most frequent response to the question asking what is going well with bedside report included the following: 'checks of intravenous medication and safety' **(assisting nursing duties),** 'introduction of oncoming staff' **(introduction of nurse/patient),** 'assessment of patient status' **(assisting nursing duties)** and 'able to see patients earlier in the shift' **(assisting nursing**

> **duties) and (introduction of nurse/patient)** ... In addition, some nurses stated that bedside report 'improves accountability' and 'increases patient involvement' **(involvement in care).** (Sand-Jecklin and Sherman 2013: 190)

Step 2: developing themes

As you read through the results of all the papers, you will identify more codes and you will begin to see how these codes come together into potential themes. It is useful to tabulate the emerging themes and the papers they have been identified in. You will find that some of the themes arise in all papers and that some arise in only a few of the papers.

There are different ways to manage this process:

- Some people 'cut and paste' the data from their papers into themes so that they capture the entire content of the results within each theme – do keep a second copy of the paper for reference if you use this approach. This can be a good way to proceed if you like to work visually. It is appropriate even in an age of technology.
- Others like to transcribe the theme onto an electronic document so that all the extracts about each theme are grouped together electronically – if you use this approach, remember to give as much detail and avoid summarizing the data so that you retain a full description.

It is advisable to keep the original documents to hand at this time – do not put them to one side as you will need to refer back to them to check for accuracy of the themes you are developing. Once you have allocated all the findings in the papers into themes, you need to merge all the data allotted to the same theme.

It is often useful to display the results of your data analysis visually on a chart such as the one presented in Table 7.1. You will then see a picture begin to emerge about the different codes and themes as they are described in your papers. Be prepared to reconsider the names of the codes and the themes and to move data around from one theme to another as your understanding of your data increases.

Step 3: naming your themes

As you continue to develop your themes, you will need to consider a provisional name for the themes as they develop. It is important to

Table 7.1 Display of qualitative themes

Author (date)	Introduction of nurse/ patient	Assisting nursing duties	Involvement in care	Enhance relationship between nurse and patient
Sand-Jecklin and Sherman (2013)	✓	✓	✓	
Jeffs et al. (2013)	✓	✓	✓	✓

emphasize that the names of the themes are provisional at this stage. As you continue to look at the results of the papers and your understanding of the data develops, you can re-name your themes as appropriate.

Step 4: comparing the themes

The next step is to revisit each theme and check two things:

- Have you got the 'best fit' name for the theme?
- Do all the individual codes fit into the theme?

Lincoln and Guba (1985: 342) describe how this 'dynamic working back and forth' gives the researcher confidence that the development of themes is robust and open to scrutiny.

It is at this point that the similarities and differences in the findings of your review will begin to emerge. Look closely at the themes you are developing and begin to consider how they are linked together. This is why it is important to keep the original documents close to hand as you may need to refer back to them to check some information or to seek further information that becomes required as your analysis progresses. If you have 'cut and pasted' the results from the original papers and grouped these together into themes, you can refer back to the original sources easily. If you have compiled the themes electronically, make sure you refer back to the original sources so that you arrive at the full meaning of the data. You will find that you have further questions that you want to ask of the papers you have and so will need ready access to them.

It is sometimes recommended that two or three people code each paper in order to generate maximum insight about the meaning of that paper. Unless you are working on a large funded project, this is not always possible; however, you might find it useful to discuss this process with your project supervisor or ask a friend or colleague to look over your ideas. If you do, remember to write this up in your methods section.

Step 5: consider the impact of poorer-quality studies on your analysis

This is where you refer back to your critical appraisal. You will give more weight to a paper that provides strong evidence than to a weaker paper, and this is why critical appraisal is important.

What is the impact of poorer-quality research in your literature review? Thomas and Harden (2008) suggest that a sensitivity analysis will help you to determine the impact of weaker studies in your literature review. Just as, in a meta-analysis, researchers sometimes do the statistics with and without the weaker studies, this is also possible within a thematic analysis. If you analyse your literature including and excluding a weaker study, you can identify the impact that the weaker study has in a particular theme. Thomas and Harden argue that, often, poorer-quality studies will simply contribute less to the ongoing analysis rather than distort it.

Step 6: consider the extent to which all your data are consistent

You might find that you have individual themes that do not support one another. The first thing to do is to consider the context of each paper from which the theme arose, together with the strengths and limitations of the research approaches undertaken. You need to return to your original critical appraisal of each paper at this point, as you need to re-assess the strength of the evidence in addressing your particular question. The rationale behind a review is that all the relevant literature is reviewed so that you can see each piece of literature in the context of the other available literature, and that differences and similarities in the results can be compared.

When you encounter literature that presents a different picture to that given by the previous literature you examined, it is important to document it carefully. Describe the differences in results and do not attempt to hide these in order to make your results appear more coherent. If all the data suggest different things, document this and say that you cannot reach firm conclusions from the data at your disposal.

You can also compare the results of research reports with non-research papers in this way, but again the contexts of both must be fully acknowledged. For example, a discussion paper by a leading expert might argue one point, but this point may not be borne out in the actual research studies that have addressed the same issues. You are likely to find research reports that contradict the opinion of an expert in the research topic area and vice versa.

Step 7: use interpretation to explain the results

Remember that this is your analysis – be creative, but ensure that you can justify the names of the themes and the inclusion of data from the original studies into those themes. At the end of this process you should have a firmed-up set of themes with names that convey the meaning of the data within them.

In summary

In this chapter, we have introduced a range of approaches for analysing data when doing a literature review. The approaches discussed are by no means exhaustive and not always specific to a particular overall method for undertaking a review. In one study, Hannes and Macaitis (2012) explored the approaches to analysis used by researchers doing different types of literature review. Hannes and Macaitis identified Noblet and Hare's meta-ethnography as the most popular method of data analysis. Thematic analysis, as described by Thomas and Harden (2008), was also popular but sometimes lacked a definite procedure. The terminology used by authors can also vary. For example, Walsh and Downe (2005) and Benza and Liamputtong (2014) describe Noblit and Hare's (1988) meta-ethnography approach as a meta-synthesis. The important point here is to be aware of the range of approaches, to identify the approach that is most appropriate for your study and to provide a clear rationale for why you chose it.

At post-graduate level, it is important to strive for a sound and rigorous methodological approach and to avoid merging approaches without a clear rationale. So, we would advise you to adhere to one of the approaches we discuss in this book.

For all approaches, you will find that when you undertake a detailed systematic analysis and synthesis of the data from your literature, your findings will be displayed in a format whereby comparisons across studies can be made more easily. This can be quantitatively, such as a meta-analysis, or qualitatively, using a form of thematic analysis. Broadly speaking, there are two possible positions from which you may approach your analysis and synthesis of literature:

- Meta-analysis or description of statistical data
- Thematic analysis of qualitative or mixed methods.

If your data are quantitative, you may consider undertaking a meta-analysis or a summary of the findings using descriptive statistics. We have referred you to further texts in order to do so. If your data are qualitative, mixed-methods in nature, or a mixture of research and other evidence, you are likely to analyse and synthesize your data using one of the approaches we have discussed in this chapter. We have provided references for the full text of the papers or books in which these approaches are discussed and we recommend that you access these when you have identified which approach to adopt. Whichever approach you use, it is important that you can describe and justify your rationale for choosing it.

With all of the approaches, undertaking a detailed analysis and synthesis enables you to see the strengths and weaknesses of studies and to highlight key findings, providing greater emphasis to the stronger studies. You can then start to develop arguments and generate critical understanding of the findings through a narrative report or section, which we will discuss in the next chapter.

Key points

- There are a wide variety of approaches to the analysis and synthesis of literature in your review
- Some use a quantitative or statistical form of data analysis
- Others use a qualitative or mixed-methods approach to data analysis
- There are differences in the approach to searching and critical appraisal when using the qualitative and mixed-methods approaches
- All of the qualitative and mixed-methods approaches use a narrative form of analysis
- It is important that you identify and justify which approach is appropriate for your study.

8

How do I write up my literature review?

In this chapter, we will discuss:

- *The overall presentation of your literature review*
- *How to present your review for publication.*

You will have now completed a comprehensive search, data extraction, critical appraisal and analysis of the data (usually research) and other evidence that constitutes your review. It is a well-established principle that research reviews are considered 'research of research' and should have the same standard of rigour as empirical research (Whittemore and Knafl 2005). Therefore, it is important that you understand that your literature review is a research study in its own right and should be presented as such. This will enable you to demonstrate that you have taken a systematic and comprehensive approach and will help you prepare your review for publication, if this is one of your aims. In some cases, students are required to submit their work in the format of a manuscript for publication in a specific journal or even to produce a number of published papers as part of their thesis. In this context, it is important that you think carefully about how to prepare the manuscript, following the author guidelines from your target journal.

You need to consider how you will present your review so that it is sufficiently succinct but demonstrates the detail with which you have engaged with the literature and undertaken the analysis and synthesis.

Most research studies are presented in the conventional style of Introduction, Methods, Results and Discussion, which is sometimes described using the acronym IMRAD (Sollaci and Pereira 2004). If you look at how other published literature reviews are presented, especially systematic reviews, you will see that they usually follow this structure, and adherence to this structure is generally agreed to be a feature of a good-quality literature review within health and social care (Aveyard 2023).

The way in which you present your review will depend on the role it plays in your post-graduate project (Table 8.1). Your review will either be a standalone project, in which the results of your literature review are the main results of your project and will summarize what we know about the review question, or your review might be supportive of a larger empirical study in which case the results will demonstrate a gap in the knowledge, thus justifying your subsequent empirical research study. As discussed previously, however, these differences tend to be subtle and what is important is that you present your review in an appropriately structured way, with reference to the IMRAD acronym as discussed above.

If the review forms the main part of your thesis, then you are likely to have a much larger word count for it than if it forms only one chapter. However, all reviews need to highlight the gaps in research evidence and the need for further research.

Reporting guidelines

The use of reporting guidelines is now a standard requirement of most academic journals for all types of submissions. Reporting guidelines provide pointers to key stages in a study or review which need to be addressed in the reporting, or writing up, of the study. One common area of confusion is to conflate a reporting guideline with the method by which the study is undertaken. Although there are similarities, the two are different: the method provides the 'recipe' by which the study is undertaken, while the reporting guideline provides the 'outline' by which the study should be reported.

For anyone undertaking a literature review, there are a number of reporting guidelines that can be used to report the study, including the PRISMA guidelines (for systematic review with or without meta-analysis and mixed-methods reviews) and the ENTREQ guidelines (for qualitative and mixed-methods reviews). These and many other specific reporting guidelines can be accessed via the EQUATOR website and provide a useful checklist for what to include in your publication. Aveyard et al. (2023)

provide an analysis of the practicalities of using a reporting guideline when you write up your study. This includes the importance of selecting the most appropriate guideline and to refrain from shoe horning a study into an inappropriate guideline.

The structure of your literature review

In the sections below, we discuss the individual sections of your literature review and the content you would be expected to include. The information provided is a guide only and you are advised to follow the specific criteria provided by your academic institution, and if you are seeking to submit your work for publication, then you must carefully follow the author guidelines for your selected journal.

Introduction and background

In your introduction, you need to explain the literature review question you are going to answer and clarify the purpose of your review and the role it plays in your project, as summarized in Table 8.1. You also need to define the key terms that you will be using. If there is a recent concept analysis of any of the key terms you are using, it would be useful to draw upon this. While it is important to explain and justify your literature review question, it is important not to answer it in your introduction. Therefore, you must avoid any reference to the papers that you have identified from your search that address your literature review question. The introduction also normally includes a concise description of what is already known about the topic, drawing upon the literature. For example, you might need to explain the epidemiology of a disease, the policy context and/or the range of services available, depending upon the topic you are focusing on. All of this information can be included in a separate background chapter in which you set the study in the context of what is already known. You may draw on this again in the discussion chapter if you are preparing a PhD thesis. We advise you to carefully check on your institution's requirements.

Methods

In your methods section, you will discuss the rationale for your chosen approach to the literature review. So, for example, if you have undertaken a systematic review with meta-analysis, you need to explain why

Table 8.1 Reflecting on the purpose of your literature review

Your literature is likely to fall into one of these categories, although sometimes the distinction might not be as clear as we have shown here	Your literature review is a standalone study. The aim of your review is to answer (or partially answer) your literature review question	Your literature review is supportive to a subsequent empirical study. The aim of your review is to identify gaps in knowledge that lead on to your empirical study

you considered this approach to be appropriate. Alternatively, if you undertook a meta-ethnographic study, you need to explain your rationale for doing this. You will then outline the steps you undertook to complete your literature review including your search strategy, data extraction, critical appraisal, analysis and synthesis. Your methods section is likely to read like a recipe – explaining exactly what you did. This helps to make the review transparent and reassures the reader that you have been comprehensive and systematic in your methods. Remember to refer directly to your literature review question. If you have more than one literature review question, you need to explain each review separately. If you have written up the methods in a separate protocol, you might consider summarizing this in your thesis but including the full protocol in an appendix.

Search strategy

Your search strategy needs to be clearly documented in your methods section so that the examiner or reader of your work could replicate it if necessary. In fact, sometimes this might be a part of the assessment strategy. You need to document all the key terms and synonyms you used, how you combined these using Boolean operators, how you used truncation and controlled subject headings. The overall aim is to demonstrate to the reader that you have included all the key terms that could be reasonably expected and that you have not omitted terms that would render your review incomplete. It is useful to include a PRISMA diagram to demonstrate the process you followed, including the total number of papers identified, how decisions were made about these papers, how many duplicates there were, how many papers you read in full, as discussed in Chapter 4.

Data extraction

The way in which you undertook data extraction needs to be documented in your methods section. You should include a copy of the data extraction tool you developed and used for your review question. You should also include a completed data extraction tool in the appendix of your literature review.

Critical appraisal

Your approach to critical appraisal should be discussed in your methods section. You should also discuss the use of any critical appraisal tools used in the study and why these were chosen. If you did not use a specific tool, you should explain your rationale for not doing so. It can be helpful to include a completed example of a critical appraisal tool in your appendix.

Analysis and synthesis

Your approach to the analysis and synthesis of literature should be described in your methods section. As we have discussed throughout this book, there are a variety of possible methods of data analysis and synthesis, and it is important that you can justify the approach you have taken and provide a rationale as to why you considered it appropriate for your study. Given the complexity of approaches and discussion of approaches, you are advised to refer directly to the original authors who developed or are developing the methods you have used for your analysis and synthesis of the literature. If you have amended the methods, then it is important to document what you have done and why.

Results

Your results need to be clearly presented, as you would expect the results of a research study to be.

It is useful to commence the presentation of your results with an overview of your papers. This can include the geographical areas they arise from, the methods they used, the dates of publication and so on.

The presentation of your results will depend on the approach you used to analyse and synthesize your literature. Results of a meta-analysis can be clearly displayed in a forest plot. Results from a qualitative or mixed-methods approach can be presented visually as a chart or matrix, but this chart/matrix also needs to be accompanied by a clear description of the data or literature you used to compile it. This should be a summary rather than a list of individual papers. Hence your chart or matrix is likely to be followed by a detailed discussion of all the themes referred to in it. Consider how the findings relate to each other and why different findings might have arisen. Different populations, contexts, interventions and methods of measurement might have affected the findings of the studies.

If you have found a variety of outcome measures that were difficult to make sense of, you need to explain how this has affected the results or findings of your review. It is useful to describe the way in which the interventions and outcome measures were different. For example, if an intervention was specialist care, then you can describe what this meant in each paper. This is important as it enables you to demonstrate your skills of critical appraisal – otherwise you are just reporting the results of the work of others in an uncritical way.

It is useful to compare and contrast the data which make up your themes, where the themes support each other (reciprocal themes) and where they do not (refutational themes). If your word count permits, it is also useful to provide a short summary of the way in which you used the critical appraisal within your analysis. You might have analysed the literature both with and without the weaker studies in order to determine the effect of including them. You may have included only the methodologically strongest studies. It is important to discuss your reasons for the decisions you made.

Discussion

The final stage of your literature review is to bring your whole project together. This involves reflecting on your results and the way you can relate these to the literature review question more broadly.

This means that you have to interpret the meaning of your results and the implications they have for your project as a whole and your area of practice where appropriate. This needs to be set in the context of the limitations of what you have done. You also need to include a discussion of how your project has contributed to knowledge and theoretical understandings. Finally, you are likely to make recommendations for future research and practice. Although you are at the end of the literature review process, it is important not to rush this final section; it is your opportunity to shine and demonstrate creativity.

The following suggested structure is a guide based on the work of Doherty and Smith (1999) and Drotar (2009) regarding how to discuss the findings of a research project. We suggest you follow this structure when writing up your discussion and attend to each of the following points:

- Statement of findings
- Strength and limitations of your study
- Discussion of your findings: linking to what is previously known on the topic
- Recommendations and implications for practice, policy or further research.

The emphasis in your discussion section will depend on whether your literature review is a standalone study – in which case your discussion will seek to summarize what you have found out about your question – or whether it is a prerequisite to a larger study – in which case you will be highlighting the gaps in knowledge and hence the need for further research (Table 8.2).

Statement of findings

The findings from your literature review should be summarized, to emphasize the new knowledge your review has generated. This should be a concise summary, rather than a repetition of the details of your results section. If possible, you should summarize your findings in one or two sentences. This is only possible at the end of a study when you have done a thorough analysis and synthesis of your literature. You will not be in a position to write a concise and accurate summary until you have completed your analysis and synthesis.

Table 8.2 Differences between the discussion section in a 'standalone' vs. 'main study' literature review

Your main project is an **empirical study** (for example, a PhD or master's-level project)	Your discussion will focus on the next stage of your project – including how your literature review has highlighted the need for further research and a gap in the knowledge related to your research question
Your main project is a **standalone literature review** (for example, a master's-level project)	Your discussion will focus on the extent to which you have been able to answer your literature review question based on the available literature

At this point, it is necessary to interpret your findings. For example, what do your findings mean in the context of what is already known? What is new about your work? Does it agree with (or contradict) what is already known? Ensure that your interpretation conveys the meaning of your findings, which you need to do in just a few sentences. You will likely require several attempts at this before you communicate succinctly the meaning of your findings. Try different ways, look objectively at the meaning of what you have written and consider whether you have captured the essence of your results in these sentences. A lack of clarity about your findings often indicates a lack of clarity about your project as a whole.

You should also comment on the methods used in the papers you reviewed, the characteristics of the groups of participants involved in the studies and what this says about the literature you included. If all of the research papers you reviewed are surveys, you might want to comment on the relevance of this to your project. Alternatively, if all the research papers were focused on the perspective of the patient or client rather than the health or social care professional, you might want to comment on that.

Some theoretical reflections are also useful. If all of the papers included in your review refer to a particular theoretical perspective, this should be commented on. For example, you might find that all your papers refer to the attachment theory of Bowlby rather than to other theories of child development.

Strengths and limitations of your study

It is important to acknowledge the strengths and limitations of your literature review. This will inform the reader of any drawbacks to your research and allows the results to be placed in context. In the same way that you critically appraised the studies upon which your literature review is based, it is also necessary to undertake a critical appraisal of your own work.

Be sure to emphasize what you have done to enhance the rigour of your study. Discuss the involvement of colleagues or your supervisor in the data selection, extraction, analysis and synthesis stages of your project if appropriate. Would additional resources have enabled you to undertake a more detailed review? For example, extra finances might have allowed you to employ the assistance of another researcher to aid you in the search, critique and bringing together of the literature.

You can also mention what you have learnt from undertaking this research process and how you would approach a similar study in the future.

Discussion of your findings

This section can be one of the most difficult to write. Up to this point, you will have followed a systematic and logical process that has resulted in the presentation of the results of your study. Now is the time for some creativity on your part and to consider what your results or findings really mean in relation to your literature review question and the purpose of your review. Discussing your findings is therefore both an art and a science.

In order to do this, you need to look at your work critically, from different perspectives and with fresh eyes. If you can take a break from your review for a few days, you might consider your findings in a different light. Talk to others about your findings and their possible implications. It might be helpful to forget the detail for a moment, and consider the most important thing that your work has demonstrated: the aspects that you would most like to share with others. This should relate to those aspects of your findings that are most important for answering your research question.

While it is important to emphasize that there is an interpretive and creative element to your literature review, you need to make clear your findings and themes you developed. Do not be tempted to exaggerate your findings so that your argument flows better. This will be spotted by those responsible for examining your work, and your findings may be discredited. If your results are inconclusive, it is important to restate this rather than try to make the results appear to show something that they do not. Be honest about what you have found; remember that finding little evidence about your literature review question is a useful finding in itself. If your literature review is a prerequisite to an empirical study, finding minimal literature provides a justification for your further research and the development of theories.

However, you do need to provide some interpretation of your findings and make your own judgement on them. There is little point to a discussion section if you merely repeat the main findings of the study and do not exercise any judgement or attempt an analysis of your findings (Skelton and Edwards 2000).

The main aim of the discussion of your themes is to focus outwards and begin to consider how the main themes you have identified relate to the wider context in which your literature review or research question is located. There are three main ways in which you can do this, by considering related research, policy or theory.

Integrating your results and discussion

If you use the IMRAD framework for the presentation of your literature review, the results and discussion will be two separate sections.

However, some researchers prefer to discuss their findings immediately after they have presented them. In this way, the theme and the discussion are read consecutively so that the reader can follow the flow of the argument. If you opt to present your results and findings this way, it is important to inform the reader that this is your intention and also to ensure that your discussion does not get 'mixed up' with your results.

Relating your themes to further research

You might consider relating your themes to research in another, related area. For example, if your literature review focused on a certain group of patients or clients, you could discuss your findings in the light of the findings of research that relate to a different group of patients or clients. If your literature review question concerned what it is like for homeless people to access medical or social care services, you might compare your findings with the experience of other 'hard to reach' groups. In order to do this, you will need to do some additional literature searches to identify papers that shed light on the topic of your literature review question in these alternative circumstances. The detail in which you do this will depend on the level at which you are studying.

Relating your themes to relevant policy

You might consider relating your themes to other policy to determine whether the findings of your review are in line with current policy. For example, if your literature review focused on the administration of medications and your results indicated that patients/clients prefer to administer their own medication while in hospital, you might compare how this finding reflects policy on the self-administration of medication.

Relating your themes to relevant theories

You might also consider relating your themes directly back to the theories you identified at the start of your project or to new theories which you have come across in your review. For example, if your review focused on what motivates people to lose weight, or to change any aspect of their behaviour, you could compare your findings against current theories of behaviour change. You could also comment on the way in which your review has highlighted assumptions or problems with existing theories.

Recommendations for further research and practice

If your literature review is a standalone review, you should be able to identify some clear recommendations for practice and further research. Remember that these have arisen from your own original work and so you can be bold about the assertions you make. It is useful to give examples from your review to illustrate why the recommendations have been made. If your results are inconclusive, then you are likely to suggest that further research is needed. It is important to consider the way in which recommendations are made, according to your level of study. Recommendations can be listed clearly as bullet points with accompanying rationale or you may consider a more in-depth approach to the presentation and discussion of your recommendations.

Dissemination and publication

One of the obvious benefits of taking a systematic approach to your literature review is the possibility that your work will be published. Presenting your review as a study in its own right will emphasize the importance of your review and any subsequent studies that follow on. Publication of your literature review will enhance the credibility of your overall project and the comments from the reviewers will provide you with an additional source of feedback. This is especially relevant for PhD candidates. If your review is published before your viva, it will be clear to your examiners that your work has already been peer reviewed. Do consider publishing guidelines such as PRISMA (prisma-statement.org) or Tong et al. (2012) for qualitative reviews when writing your review for publication. The level of rigour with which you have approached your review will indicate where your review can be published. The data extraction tool we provided in Chapter 5 on the management of pleural effusion (Table 5.2) was submitted for publication by the Cochrane Collaboration (Clive et al. 2013). This was because it entailed a highly rigorous method, incorporating a team of reviewers at different stages of the project. The other example in Chapter 5 on the perception of services by people experiencing a life-limiting illness (Table 5.3) was submitted to a specialist palliative care journal. The rigour of this study was commented on as there was only one reviewer involved in the review process.

As a general principle, it is advisable to consult the publication guidelines for any journal to which you might submit. We advise that you do this at your earliest opportunity as you can then write with the intention of publishing in this journal. Remember that different journals accept different types of literature review. The extent to which you can show rigour in the methods undertaken in your review will affect your chances of publication. Those journals with the highest impact are likely to require that you have searched on multiple databases, involved colleagues or peers in different stages of the review as discussed in Chapters 4 and 5, and presented a PRISMA checklist to demonstrate that you have followed the recognized stages of a systematic review. In addition to rigour in the methods used, you also need to demonstrate the impact and usefulness of the review, so the discussion section is vital.

Above all, you need to be concise in your presentation. Journal papers are often limited to 3,000–5,000 words. Many are not able to print multiple tables but this might be possible in online editions. You may have to edit and summarize the main findings of your review but you can refer the reader to the full version of your project or thesis for further information.

Practical ways to enhance the presentation of your literature review

There are some straightforward and practical ways that you can enhance the presentation of your work. This might sound obvious, but clearly presented work will make it easier for your examiner to award you marks. The following are some tips to help you with your presentation:

- Ask a friend or colleague to proofread your work
- Concentrate on checking for typos
- Return to your work after a break and read it again with fresh eyes
- Make good use of headings and tables
- Make sure all your references are complete.

In summary

Remember that a literature review is a study in its own right and you should usually present it as such, according to the standard scientific structure of IMRAD. Presenting your review according to this structure will also enable you to prepare your work for publication as most journals will require this structure. When you write up your methods, you need to write succinctly while not losing the detail and complexity with which you undertook your review. Your results section should be presented as a meta-analysis or use a theme-based approach, with a justification for the approach you took. Your discussion needs to relate your main findings to relevant research, theories or policies. Finally, remember to summarize the extent to which your review has answered your research question or paved the way for your subsequent larger empirical study.

Key points

- Your literature review should normally be written up using the standard scientific structure, IMRAD
- You need to give clear and succinct details about the method you undertook in your literature review, including how you searched, extracted data, and appraised and analysed your literature
- Ensure your discussion is an accurate reflection of the results
- Summarize your main findings in the discussion section, but briefly!
- Acknowledge the strengths and limitations of your review
- Discuss your findings in relation to clinical practice, research, policies or theories
- Discuss any unanswered questions and recommendations for future research.

Appendix

Data Extraction form

Name of reviewer: Nancy	Date of data extraction: 20/8/14	Study ID: –

Study Details:

Lead Author Ba	
Year 2013	
Country (ies)	CHINA.
Start of recruitment	Dec 2008
End of recruitment	Dec 2011
Intended duration of follow up for each patient (months)- please state maximum	
Number of recruiting centres:	? 1
If >1 recruiting centres, is the trial cluster randomised?	Yes / No / (NA)
Type of report: (F=full text; A=abstract; U=unpublished)	F
Language	English.
What is the study evaluating? (A= pleurodesis agent; B= mode of admin of pleurodesis; C= other method to optimise pleurodesis; D = IPC)	C

Eligibility Checklist:

INCLUSION CRITERIA	Answer to all must be yes
Is the study population >16 years of age?	✓
Does the study population have symptomatic pleural effusion from an underlying malignant process?	✓
Is the trial an RCT or randomised cross over trial?	✓

EXCLUSION CRITERIA	Answer to all must be no
Does the study include patients with both malignant and non malignant disease, with no clear distinction between the groups in the results section?	No
Is the study evaluating the effect of a drug administered via a method other than the intra-pleural route?	No
Does the study include effusions in a number of different body cavities (eg peritoneum, pericardium), with no distinction between the groups in the results section?	No

Will you continue with data extraction? (Yes) No

If no, please state reason:

Details of the intervention:

Common treatment for all groups (therefore not under comparison)	Drainage of Pleural effusion using Hassan trocar.		
Group	**1**	**2**	**3**
Description of intervention	DW – Distilled water 48°C	Physiological Saline + cisplatinum	
Dose	500 mls 48°C	500 mls + 70mg cisplat 48°C	
Number of doses given & frequency	① x3 after tube placement ② ICU ③ 2nd + 4th day		
Mode of administration	IP	IP	
Number of patients randomised	12	11	
Number lost to follow up & reasons	0	0	
Which group was used as the control? (tick one)		? ✓	
How did you decide which was the control group? (tick one)	Assumed by data extractor ☑ Stated in paper ☐		

Patient characteristics:

Inclusion criteria	MPE by CXR or CT ≥18 yrs ~~Limited encapsulated PE~~ 1° cancer.	
Exclusion criteria	THORACOTOMY LIMITED ENCAPSULATED PE EXTENSIVE PLEURAL ADHESIONS	
Type of cancer (A= all; B=meso; C= lung; D=breast/gynae; E=GI; F=urol/renal; G=other (please specify))	A	
Other potential confounding variables identified? (eg steroid, NSAIDS, trapped lung, or others.....)	Yes / (No)	If yes, please specify:
Were the groups broadly similar at baseline? Eg Age, Sex, WHO PS, Number with trapped lung	Yes / No ? If no, please specify: ALL LISTED TOGETHER.	

Study aims:

Relevant primary outcome(s)	Description	How was it measured?	Time point(s) at which it was measured?	Comments
1	CR	UNKNOWN	UNCLEAR.	NOT REALLY EXPLAINED.
2				

Relevant secondary outcome(s)	Description	How was it measured?	Time point(s) at which it was measured?	Comments
1	P-S KARNOFSKY →	SCALE	AFTER Rx ?	
2				
3				
4				
5				
6				
7				
8				
9				

Study Quality (please refer to this when completing the risk of bias table)

Was a power calculation performed?	Yes / No [circled: No]
Was the study analysed on an intention to treat basis?	Yes / No / Unsure [circled: Unsure] BUT ALL INCLUDED
Method of randomisation (eg telephone, envelopes...)	UNKNOWN
Is there substantial missing outcome data? (Eg withdrawals/loss to FU. Are reasons given for withdrawals?)	Yes / No / unsure [circled: No] If yes, please specify:
Were all the aims of the study reported on?	Yes / No / Unsure [circled: Yes; Unsure crossed out]
Any specific points or issues about the study's quality?	VERY POOR REPORTING EVEN WHAT CR IS AND WHEN MEASURED – ? EXCLUDE.

Results: Please insert ABSOLUTE NUMBERS, not %

PLEURODESIS

Timepoint	Group	Pleurodesis success	Pleurodesis failure	Total	Are patients who have died prior to this timepoint included as a success or a failure?*	Method used to define pleurodesis success**
?	1	10	2	12	NA	? NO FLUID ON X-RAY.
	2	9	2	11	NA	
	3					
	1					
	2					
	3					
	1					
	2					
	3					

* If the data is available, patients who die prior to the timepoint being evaluated should still be included for the analysis (ie if they die with no symptomatic recurrence of effusion, this is a success).
** KEY: A= radiological resolution; B= need for repeat pleural procedure; C= as measured by trial investigators; D= minimal drainage from IPC & radiographic evidence of no significant residual collection; E= other (please specify)

MORTALITY

Timepoint	Group	Number of patients alive	Number of patients dead	Total
	1			
	2			
	3			
	1			
	2			
	3			
	1			
	2			
	3			

MEDIAN SURVIVAL

Group 1				Group 2				Group 3			
n	Median	SD	CI	n	Median	SD	CI	n	Median	SD	CI
12	13m	(30-30m)		11	12.9	4-26m					

SYMPTOM SCALE -Please include quality of life, pain and breathlessness scales or any other symptom scores. If reported, please also include any score of patient acceptability of the intervention.

1. Which scale? KARNOFSKY .

		Baseline				Follow up				Change			
Time point	Group	n	Mean	SD	CI	n	Mean	SD	CI	n	Mean	SD	CI
?	1	12	54	?±40%		12	77.2	?		12	23.2		
	2	11	54.4	?		11	77.5	?		11	23.1		
	3												
	1												
	2												
	3												
	1												
	2												
	3												

2. Which scale? ______________

		Baseline				Follow up				Change			
Time point	Group	n	Mean	SD	CI	n	Mean	SD	CI	n	Mean	SD	CI
	1												
	2												
	3												
	1												
	2												
	3												
	1												
	2												
	3												

3. Which scale? ______________

		Baseline				Follow up				Change			
Time point	Group	n	Mean	SD	CI	n	Mean	SD	CI	n	Mean	SD	CI
	1												
	2												
	3												
	1												
	2												
	3												
	1												
	2												
	3												

4. Which scale? ______________

		Baseline				Follow up				Change			
Time point	Group	n	Mean	SD	CI	n	Mean	SD	CI	n	Mean	SD	CI
	1												
	2												
	3												
	1												
	2												
	3												
	1												
	2												
	3												

DURATION OF INPATIENT STAY (if available)

Timepoint	Group	n	Mean	SD	95% CI
Randomisation to discharge	1				
	2				
	3				
	1				
	2				
	3				

COSTS (if available)

Timepoint	Group	n	Mean	SD	95% CI
	1				
	2				
	3				
	1				
	2				
	3				

ADVERSE EVENTS/ COMPLICATIONS FROM THE INTERVENTION:

Event	Group	Number effected	Number not effected	Total	Comments
	1				
	2				
	3				
	1				
	2				
	3				
	1				
	2				
	3				
	1				
	2				
	3				

Risk of bias tool:

Domain	Description and support for judgement (PLEASE FILL THIS IN!!!)	Review authors judgment HIGH= High risk of bias LOW= low risk of bias
Sequence generation - Low risk of bias (any truly random process, eg random number table; computer generated) - High risk of bias (any non-random process, eg odd or even DOB; hospital or clinic record number) - Unclear risk of bias: the trial may or may not be free of bias	NOT STATED	Was the allocation sequence adequately generated? HIGH / LOW / UNCLEAR
Allocation concealment Could the allocation could have been foreseen prior to or during recruitment? - Low risk of bias (e.g. telephone or central randomisation; consecutively numbered sealed opaque envelopes) - High risk of bias (open random allocation; unsealed or non-opaque envelopes, alternation; date of birth) - Unclear risk of bias- the trial may or may not be free of bias	NOT ENOUGH INFO	Was allocation adequately concealed? HIGH / LOW / UNCLEAR
Blinding of participants, personnel and outcome assessors - Low risk of bias: Blinded and method used for blinding described - Unknown risk: if they stated that they were blinded, but did not describe how it was achieved. - High risk of bias: Unblinded	NONE STATED.	Was knowledge of the allocated intervention adequately prevented during the study? HIGH / LOW / UNCLEAR
Incomplete outcome data - Include whether study analysed on an intention to treat basis - Is these lots of missing outcome data? (Eg withdrawls/ loss to FU. Are reasons given for withdrawls?)	ALL THERE	Were incomplete outcome data adequately addressed? HIGH / LOW / UNCLEAR
Selective outcome reporting - Low risk of bias: all outcomes pre-defined and reported, or all clinically relevant and expected outcomes were reported. - Uncertain risk: Unclear whether all pre-defined and clinically relevant were reported. - High risk of bias: one or more clinically relevant and reasonably expected outcomes were not reported, and data on these outcomes were likely to have been recorded.	ALL THERE	Are reports of the study free of suggestion of selective outcome reporting? HIGH / LOW / UNCLEAR
Other sources of bias - Low risk of bias: the trial appears to be free of other bias, eg industry bias, academic bias) - Uncertain risk of bias: Unclear if other sources of bias - High risk of bias: Other factors in that could put trial at risk of bias (for example, for-profit involvement, authors have conducted trials on the same topic). **** Also comment here on** • method used to define pleurodesis • inc/exc patients with trapped lung	NO DEFINITION OF OUTCOME - CR NO TIMINGS NO RANDOMISATION METHOD ? EXCLUDE	Was the study apparently free of other problems that could put it at a high risk of bias? HIGH / LOW / UNCLEAR

References

Akoberg, A.K. (2005) Understanding randomised controlled trials, *Archives of Diseases in Childhood*, 90 (8): 840–844.

Alzyood, M., Jackson, D., Brooke, J. and Aveyard, H. (2018) An integrative review exploring the perceptions of patients and healthcare professionals towards patient involvement in promoting hand hygiene compliance in the hospital setting, *Journal of Clinical Nursing*, 27 (7/8): 1329–1345.

Alzyood, M., Jackson, D., Brooke, J. and Aveyard, H. (2020) Use of focus group data from countries with linguistic differences: translation, analysis and presentation, *Nurse Researcher*, 28 (1): 17–24.

Arksey, H. and O'Malley, L. (2005) Scoping studies: towards a methodological framework, *International Journal of Social Research Methodology*, 8 (1): 19–32.

Aromataris, E., Fernandez, R., Godfrey, C., Holly, C., Khalil, H. and Tungpunkom, P. (2014) Methodology for JBI umbrella reviews, *Faculty of Science, Medicine and Health Papers*, A: 3344 [https://ro.uow.edu.au/smhpapers/3344].

Atkins, S., Lewin, S., Smith, H., Engel, M., Fretheim, A. and Volmink, J. (2008) Conducting a meta-ethnography of qualitative literature: lessons learnt, *BMC Medical Research Methodology*, 8: 21 [https://doi.org/10.1186/1471-2288-8-21].

Aveyard, H. (2023) *Doing a Literature Review in Health and Social Care*. Maidenhead: Open University Press.

Aveyard, H. and Bradbury-Jones, C. (2019) An analysis of current practice in undertaking literature reviews: a focussed mapping review and synthesis, *BMC Medical Research Methodology*, 19: 105 [https://doi.org/10.1186/s12874-019-0751-7].

Aveyard, H. and Neale, J. (2009) Critical incident technique, in J. Neale (ed.) *Research Methods for Health and Social Care*. London: Palgrave Macmillan.

Aveyard, H., Bradbury-Jones, C., Ring, N. and Flemming, K. (2023) Which reporting guideline should I use and why?, *Journal of Clinical Nursing*, 32 (9/10): e15–e16.

Aveyard, H., Farquar, M. and Preston, N. (2026) *How to Read and Critique Research*, 2nd edition. London: Sage.

Barratt, H., Campbell, M., Moore, L., Zwarenstein, M. and Bower, P. (2016) Randomised controlled trials of complex interventions and large-scale transformation of services, in R. Raine, R. Fitzpatrick, H. Barratt, G. Bevan, N. Black, R. Boaden et al., *Challenges, Solutions and Future Directions in the Evaluation of Service Innovations in Health Care and Public Health.* Health Services and Delivery Research, No. 4.16. Essay 2 [https://www.ncbi.nlm.nih.gov/books/NBK361251/; accessed September 2020].

Barroso, J., Gollop, C.J., Sandelowski, M., Meynell, J., Pearce, P.F. and Collins, L.J. (2003) The challenge of searching for and retrieving qualitative studies, *Western Journal of Nursing Research*, 25 (2): 153–178.

Bartoli, D., Lombard, E., Trotta, F., Macripo, S., Pucciarelli, G. and Francesco, P. (2025) Training and support needs in transitional care from hospital to home of the health care professional-caregiver-stroke survivor triad: a meta-synthesis study, *Journal of Clinical Nursing*, 34 (2): 625–661.

Bates, M.J. (1989) The design of browsing and berry picking techniques for the online search interface, *Online Review*, 13: 407–423.

Beck, C.T. (2009) Critiquing qualitative research, *AORN Journal*, 90 (4): 543–544.

Bench, S., Stayt, L., Shah, A., Dhiman, P. and Czuber-Dochan, W. (2021) Prevalence and experience of fatigue in survivors of critical illness: a mixed-methods systematic review, *Anaesthesia*, 76 (9): 1233–1244.

Benza, S. and Liamputtong, P. (2014) Pregnancy, childbirth and motherhood: a meta-synthesis of the lived experience of immigrant women, *Midwifery*, 30 (6): 575–584.

Betrán, A.P., Say, L., Gülmezoglu, A.M., Allen, T. and Hampson, L. (2005) Effectiveness of different databases in identifying studies for systematic reviews: experience from the WHO systematic review of maternal morbidity and mortality, *BMC Medical Research Methodology*, 5 (1): 6 [https://doi.org/10.1186/1471-2288-5-6].

Bettany-Saltikov, J. (2012) *How to Do a Systematic Literature Review in Nursing.* Maidenhead: Open University Press.

Bhaskar, R. (1978) *A Realist Theory of Science.* Hassocks: Harvester Press.

Bondas, T. and Hall, E.O.C. (2007) Challenges in approaching metasynthesis research, *Qualitative Health Research*, 17 (1): 113–121.

Booth, A. (2008) Unpacking your literature search toolbox: on search styles and tactics, *Health Information and Libraries Journal*, 25 (4): 313–317.

Booth, A. (2010) How much searching is enough? Comprehensive versus optimal retrieval for technology assessments, *International Journal of Technology Assessments in Health Care*, 26 (4): 431–435.

Booth, A. (2019) Harnessing energies, resolving tensions: acknowledging a dual heritage for qualitative evidence synthesis, *Qualitative Health Research*, 29 (1): 18–31.

Booth, A. and Carroll, C. (2015) Systematic searching for theory to inform systematic reviews: is it feasible or desirable, *Health Information Libraries Research*, 32 (3): 220–235.

Borgerson, K. (2009) Valuing evidence: bias and the evidence hierarchy of evidence-based medicine, *Perspectives in Biology and Medicine*, 52 (2): 218–233.

Bradshaw, A. (2015) Shaping the future of nursing: developing an appraisal framework for public engagement with nursing policy reports, *Nursing Inquiry*, 22 (1): 74–83.

Braun, V., and Clarke, V. (2006) Using thematic analysis in psychology, *Qualitative Research in Psychology*, 3(2), 77–101.

Brenan, V., Mio, M. and Palese, A. (2020) Nursing handovers and patient safety: findings from an umbrella review, *Journal of Advanced Nursing*, 76 (4): 927–928.

Britten, N., Campbell, R., Pope, C., Donovan, J., Morgan, M. and Pill, R. (2002) Using meta-ethnography to synthesise qualitative research: a worked example, *Journal of Health Services Research and Policy*, 7 (4): 209–215.

Brouwers, M.C., Kho, M.E., Browman, G.P., Burgers, J.S., Cluzeau, F., Feder, G. et al. (2010) AGREE II: advancing guideline development, reporting and evaluation in health care, *Canadian Medical Association Journal*, 182 (18): E839–E842.

Burls, A. (2009) *What is Critical Appraisal?* What is ...? series. Newmarket: Haywood Medical Communications.

Campbell, M., McKenzie, J.E., Sowden, A., Katikireddi, S.V., Brennan, S.E., Ellis, S. et al. (2020) Synthesis without meta-analysis (SWiM) in systematic reviews: reporting guideline, *British Medical Journal*, 368: l6890 [https://doi.org/10.1136/bmj.l6890].

Campbell, R., Pound, P., Morgan, M., Daker-White, G., Britten, P., Pill, R. et al. (2011) Evaluating meta-ethnography: systematic analysis and synthesis of qualitative research, *Health Technology Assessment*, 15 (43): 1–164.

Carroll, C., Booth, A. and Lloyd-Jones, M. (2012) Should we exclude inadequately reported studies from qualitative systematic reviews? An evaluation of sensitivity analysis in two case study reviews, *Qualitative Health Research*, 22 (10): 1425–1434.

Centre for Reviews and Dissemination (2008) *Systematic Reviews: CRD's Guidance for Undertaking Reviews in Health Care.* York: University of York [https://www.york.ac.uk/media/crd/Systematic_Reviews.pdf].

Chandler, J. and Hopewell, S. (2013) Cochrane methods: twenty years experience in developing systematic review methods, *Systematic Reviews*, 2: 76 [https://doi.org/10.1186/2046-4053-2-76].

Chapman, A.L., Morgan, L.C. and Gartlehner, G. (2009) Semi-automating the manual literature search for systematic reviews increases efficiency, *Health Information and Libraries Journal*, 27 (1): 22–27.

Chaves-Montero, A., Blanco-Miguel, P. and Ríos-Vizcaíno, B. (2025) Analysis of the predictors and consequential factors of emotional exhaustion among social workers: a systematic review, *Healthcare*, 13: 552 [https://doi.org/10.3390/healthcare13050552].

Choi, G. and Kang, H. (2023) Introduction to umbrella reviews as a useful evidence-based practice, *Journal of Lipid and Atherosclerosis*, 12 (1): 3–11.

Citrome, L., Moss, S.V. and Graf, C. (2009) How to search and harvest the medical literature: let the citations come to you, and how to proceed when they do, *International Journal of Clinical Practice*, 63 (11): 1565–1570.

Cleary, M., Horsfall, J. and Hayter, M. (2014) Data collection and sampling in qualitative research: does size matter?, *Journal of Advanced Nursing*, 70 (3): 473–475.

Clive, A., Bhatnagar, R., Preston, N.J., Jones, H.E. and Maskell, N. (2013) Interventions for the management of malignant pleural effusions, *Cochrane Database of Systematic Reviews*, 5: CD010529 [https://doi.org/10.1002/14651858.CD010529].

Cochrane, A.L. (1972) *Effectiveness and efficiency: Random reflections on health services*. London: Nuffield Provincial Hospitals Trust [https://www.nuffieldtrust.org.uk/research/effectiveness-and-efficiency-random-reflections-on-health-services].

Cochrane, A.L. (1979) 1931–1971: Critical review, with particular reference to the medical profession, in *Medicines for the Year 2000*. London: Office of Health Economics.

Cooke, A., Smith, D. and Booth, A. (2012) Beyond PICO: the SPIDER tool for qualitative evidence synthesis, *Qualitative Health Research*, 22 (10): 1435–1443.

Cooper, C., Booth, A., Varley Campbell. J., Britten, N. and Garside, R. (2018) Defining the process to literature searching in systematic reviews: a literature review of guidance and supporting studies, *BMC Medical Research Methodology*, 18: 85 [https://doi.org/10.1186/s12874-018-0545-3].

Cottrell, S. (2011) *Critical Thinking Skills*. London: Palgrave Macmillan.

Coughlan, M., Cronin, P. and Ryan, F. (2007) Step by step guide to critiquing research. Part 1: quantitative research, *British Journal of Nursing*, 16 (11): 658–663.

Couto, C., Prata, A.P., Souto, S.P., Machado, J. and Viana, C.R. (2025) Nurse and midwife interventions to protect, promote and support breastfeeding: an umbrella review, *Midwifery*, 144: 104337 [https://doi.org/10.1016/j.midw.2025.104337].

Damarell, R., Morgan, D. and Tieman, J. (2020) General practitioner strategies for managing patients with multiple morbidity: a systematic review and thematic synthesis of qualitative research, *BMC Family Practice*, 21: 131 [https://doi.org/10.1186/s12875-020-01197-8].

Darukaradhya, T.B. and Krishnamurthy, J. (2025) Modifying non-communicable disease behaviours through effective health communication and behaviour change: a systematic review, *Preventive Medicine Research and Reviews*, 2 (1): 24–39.

DeMars, M. and Perruso, C. (2022) MeSH and text-word search strategies: precision, recall and their implication for library instruction, *Journal of the Medical Library Association*, 110 (1): 23–33.

Denzin, N.K. and Lincoln, P. (1994) *Handbook of Qualitative Research.* London: Sage.

Dewey. J. (1938) *Logic: The Theory of Enquiry.* New York: Longman Green.

Dixon-Woods, M., Agarwal, S., Jones, D., Young, B. and Sutton, A. (2005) Synthesising qualitative and quantitative evidence: a review of possible methods, *Journal of Health Services Research and Policy,* 10 (1): 45–53.

Dixon-Woods, M., Cavers, D. and Agarwal, S. et al. (2006) Conducting a critical interpretive synthesis of the literature on access to healthcare by vulnerable groups, *BMC Research Methodology,* 6: 35 [https://doi.org/10.1186/1471-2288-6-35].

Dixon-Woods, M., Sutton, A., Shaw, R., Miller, T., Smith, J., Young, B. et al. (2007) Appraising qualitative research for inclusion in systematic reviews: a quantitative and qualitative comparison of three methods, *Journal of Health Service Research Policy,* 12 (1): 42–47.

Dodd, S.R., Payne, S.A., Preston, N.J. and Walshe, C.E. (2020) Understanding the outcomes of supplementary support services in palliative care for older people: a scoping review and mapping exercise, *Journal of Pain and Symptom Management,* 60 (2): 449–459.

Doherty, M. and Smith, R. (1999) The case for structuring the discussion of scientific papers, *British Medical Journal,* 318: 1224 [https://doi.org/10.1136/bmj.318.7193.1224].

Drotar, D. (2009) Editorial: How to write an effective results and discussion for *Journal of Paediatric Psychology, Journal of Paediatric Psychology,* 34 (4): 330–343.

Duffy, S. and Lefebvre, C. (2023) Peer reviewing search strategies, in *SuRe Info: Summarized Research in Information Retrieval for HTA* [https://sites.google.com/york.ac.uk/sureinfo/home/peer-reviewing-search-strategies; last updated 31 March 2023].

Dunleavy, L., Walshe, C., Oriani, A. and Preston, N. (2018) Using the 'Social Marketing Mix Framework' to explore recruitment barriers and facilitators in palliative care randomised controlled trials? A narrative synthesis review, *Palliative Medicine,* 32 (5): 990–1009.

Emerson, J.D., Burdick, E., Hoaglin, D.C., Mosteller, F. and Chalmers, T.C. (1990) An empirical study of the possible relation of treatment differences to quality scores in controlled randomized clinical trials, *Controlled Clinical Trials,* 11 (5): 339–352.

Fawcett, J. (2005) Criteria for the evaluation of theory, *Nursing Science Quarterly,* 18 (2): 131–135.

Fernández-Basanta, S., Coronado, C. and Movilla-Fernández, M.J. (2020) Multicultural coping experiences of parents following perinatal loss: a meta-ethnographic synthesis, *Journal of Advanced Nursing,* 76 (1): 9–21.

Fineout-Overholt, E. and Johnston, L. (2005) Teaching EBP: asking searchable, answerable clinical questions, *World Views on Evidence-Based Nursing*, 2 (3): 157–160.

Finfgeld, D. (1999) Courage as a process of pushing beyond the struggle, *Qualitative Health Research*, 9 (6): 803–814.

Finfgeld-Connett, D. (2014) Intimate partner abuse among older women: qualitative systematic review, *Clinical Nursing Research*, 23 (6): 664–683.

Finfgeld-Connett, D. and Johnson, E.D. (2013) Literature search strategies for conducting knowledge-building and theory-generating qualitative systematic reviews, *Journal of Advanced Nursing*, 69 (1): 194–204.

Flemming, K. (2010) Synthesis of quantitative and qualitative research: an example using critical interpretive synthesis, *Journal of Advanced Nursing*, 66 (1): 201–217.

Flemming, K., Graham, H., Heirs, M., Fox, D. and Sowden, A. (2013) Smoking in pregnancy: a systematic review of qualitative research of women who commence pregnancy as smokers, *Journal of Advanced Nursing*, 69 (5): 1023–1036.

Forde-Johnson, C. (2020) *Nurse-patient interaction and the use of electronic records*, PhD work in progress, Oxford Brookes University, Oxford.

Forde-Johnson, C., Butcher, D. and Aveyard, H. (2023) An integrative review exploring the impact of Electronic Health Records (EHR) on the quality of nurse-patient interactions and communication, *Journal of Advanced Nursing*, 79 (1): 48–67.

Fothergill, L., Hayes, N., Latham, Y., Hamilton, J., Ahmed, S. and Holland. C. (2025) Understanding how, for whom and under what circumstances telecare can support independence in community-dwelling older adults: a realist review, *BMC Geriatrics*, 25: 59 [https://doi.org/10.1186/s12877-024-05650-6].

Frie, K., Hartmann-Boyce, J., Pilbeam, C., Jebb, S. and Aveyard, P. (2020) Analysing self-regulatory behaviours in response to daily weighing: a think-aloud study with follow-up interviews, *Psychology and Health*, 35 (1): 16–35.

Gilbert, R., Salanti, G., Harden, M. and See, S. (2005) Infant sleeping position and the sudden infant death syndrome: systematic review of observational studies and historical review of recommendations 1940–2002, *International Journal of Epidemiology*, 34 (4): 874–887.

Giles, T.M. and Hall, K.L. (2014) Qualitative systematic review: the unique experiences of the nurse-family member when a loved one is admitted with a critical illness, *Journal of Advanced Nursing*, 70 (7): 1451–1464.

Glaser, B.G. and Strauss, A.L. (1967) The constant comparative method of qualitative analysis, in *The Discovery of Grounded Theory*. Chicago, IL: Aldine.

Glenton, C., Colvin, C.J., Carlsen, B., Swartz, A., Lewin, S., Noyes, J. et al. (2013) Barriers and facilitators to the implementation of lay health worker programmes to improve access to maternal and child health:

qualitative evidence synthesis, *Cochrane Database of Systematic Reviews*, 2: CD010414 [https://doi.org/10.1002/14651858.CD010414.pub2].

Gotzsche, P.C. and Nielsen, M. (2011) Screening for breast cancer with mammography, *Cochrane Database of Systematic Reviews*, 1: CD001877 [https://doi.org/10.1002/14651858.CD001877.pub4].

Grant, M.J. and Booth, A. (2009) A typology of reviews: an analysis of 14 review types and associated methodologies, *Health Information and Libraries Journal*, 26 (2): 91–108.

Greenhalgh, T. (2014) @trishgreenhalgh, on Twitter, 3–5 May.

Greenhalgh, T. and Peacock, R. (2005) Effectiveness and efficiency of search methods in systematic reviews of complex evidence: audit of primary sources, *British Medical Journal*, 331 (7524): 1064–1065.

Greenhalgh, T., Robert, G., Macfarlane, F., Bate, P., Kyriakidou, O. and Peacock, R. (2005) Storylines of research in diffusion of innovation: a meta-narrative approach to systematic review, *Social Science and Medicine*, 61 (2): 417–430.

Greenhalgh, T., Kristjansson, E. and Robinson, V. (2007) Realist review to understand the efficacy of school feeding programmes, *British Medical Journal*, 335 (7625): 858–861.

Grover, S., Sandhu, P., Nijjar, G.S., Percival, A., Chudyk, A.M., Liang, J. et al. (2023) Older adults and social prescribing experience, outcomes, and processes: a meta-aggregation systematic review, *Public Health*, 218: 197–207.

Hannes, K. and Lockwood, C. (2011) Pragmatism as the philosophical foundation for the Joanna Briggs meta-aggregative approach to qualitative evidence synthesis, *Journal of Advanced Nursing*, 67 (7): 1632–1642.

Hannes, K. and Macaitis, K. (2012) A move to more systematic and transparent approaches in qualitative evidence synthesis: update on a review of published papers, *Qualitative Research*, 12 (4): 402–442.

Harden, A. (2007) *Does study quality matter in systematic reviews which include qualitative research?* Paper presented at the XV Cochrane Collaboration Colloquium, Sao Paulo, Brazil, 23–27 October [https://abstracts.cochrane.org/2007-sao-paulo/does-study-quality-matter-systematic-reviews-which-include-qualitative-research].

Harden, A. and Thomas, J. (2005) Methodological issues in combining diverse study types in systematic reviews, *International Journal of Social Research Methodology*, 8 (3): 257–271.

Harden, A., Garcia, J., Oliver, S., Rees, R., Shepherd, J., Brunton, G. et al. (2004) Applying systematic review methods to studies of people's views: an example from public health, *Journal of Epidemiology and Community Health*, 58 (9): 794–800.

Harden, A., Brunton, G., Fletcher, A. and Oakley, A. (2006) *Young people, pregnancy and social exclusion: a systematic synthesis of research evidence to identify effective, appropriate and promising approaches for prevention and support*, EPPI Report, Social Science Research Unit,

Institute of Education, University of London [https://eppi.ioe.ac.uk/cms/Portals/0/PDF%20reviews%20and%20summaries/pregnancy_social_exclusion.pdf?ver=2006-04-24-140619-143].

Harris, J., Haltbakk, J. and Dunning, T., Austrheim, G., Kirkevold, M., Johnson, M. et al. (2019) How patient and community involvement in diabetes research influences health outcomes: a realist review, *Health Expectations*, 22 (5): 907–920.

Hastings, B.J. (2025) Guidance for successful healthcare transformation: a systematic review of change management practices and outcomes, *Australian Journal of Management*, 50 (3): 985–1005.

Hawker, S., Payne, S., Kerr, C., Hardey, M. and Powell, J. (2002) Appraising the evidence: reviewing disparate data systematically, *Qualitative Health Research*, 12 (9): 1284–1299.

Henry, C., Eheroma, A. and Filoche, S. (2020) Barriers to seeking consultation for abnormal uterine bleeding: a systematic review of qualitative research, *BMC Women's Health*, 20: 123 [https://doi.org/10.1186/s12905-020-00986-8].

Higgins, J P.T., Thomas, J., Chandler, J., Cumpston, M., Li, T., Page, M.J. and Welch, V.A. (eds.) (2024) *Cochrane Handbook for Systematic Reviews of Interventions*, version 6.5 [https://www.cochrane.org/authors/handbooks-and-manuals/handbook; last updated 22 August 2024].

Hooley, R.L., Payne, S., Begovic, D., Correa-Morales, J.E., Harding, A., Hasselaar, J. et al. (2024) Collaboration, coordination and communication as facilitators of transitions for patients with advanced cancer: a scoping review linked to the Pal-Cycles project. *BMC Palliative Care*, 23: 204 [https://doi.org/10.1186/s12904-024-01510-7].

Hoppe, D.J., Schemitsch, E.H., Morshed, S., Tornetta, P., III, and Bhandari, M. (2009) Hierarchy of evidence: where observational studies fit in and why we need them, *Journal of Bone and Joint Surgery*, 91 (suppl. 3): 2–9.

Jagosh, J. (2019) Realist synthesis for public health: building an ontologically deep understanding of how programs work, for whom, and in which contexts, *Annual Review of Public Health*, 40: 361–372.

Jakimowicz, S., Stirling, C. and Duddle, M. (2015) An investigation into factors that impact patients' subjective experience of nurse led clinics: a qualitative systematic review, *Journal of Clinical Nursing*, 24 (1/2): 19–33.

Jeffs, L., Acott, A., Simpson, E., Campbell, H., Irwin, T., Lo, J. et al. (2013) The value of bedside shift reporting, *Journal of Nursing Care Quality*, 28 (3): 226–232.

Jensen, L.A. and Allen, M.N. (1996) Meta-synthesis of qualitative findings, *Qualitative Health Research*, 6 (4): 553–560.

Joanna Briggs Institute (2014) *Reviewers' Manual.* Adelaide: University of Adelaide.

Jurd, C. and Barr, J. (2024) Leadership factors for cardiopulmonary resuscitation for clinicians in-hospital; behaviours, skills and strategies: a systematic review and synthesis without meta-analysis, *Journal of Clinical Nursing*, 33 (10): 3844–3853.

Just, M.L. (2012) Is literature search training for medical students and residents effective? A literature review, *Journal of the Medical Library Association*, 100 (4): 270–276.

Katrak, P., Bialocerkowski, A.E., Massy-Westropp, N., Kumar, S. and Grimmer, K.A. (2004) A systematic review of the content of critical appraisal tools, *BMC Medical Research Methodology*, 4: 22 [https://doi.org/10.1186/1471-2288-4-22].

Kuhn, T.S. (1962) *The Structure of Scientific Revolutions*. Chicago, IL: University of Chicago Press.

Labrague, L.J. and Cayaban, A.R. (2025) Association between patient safety culture and missed nursing care in healthcare settings: a systematic review and meta-analysis, *Journal of Advanced Nursing*, 81 (11): 7992–8004.

Langenhoff, J.M. and Schoones, J.W. (2011) Letter to the editor: 'Risk factors for bladder cancer: challenges for conducting a literature search using PubMed', *Perspectives in Health Information Management*, 8 (Fall): 1g [https://pmc.ncbi.nlm.nih.gov/articles/PMC3193512/].

Lascelles, K.M., Davey, Z., Jackson, D. and Aveyard, H. (2024) Experiences and needs of adult informal carers of adults at risk of suicide: a systematic review with mixed methods analysis, *Journal of Advanced Nursing*, 80: 1686–1718.

Law, M., Stewart, D., Pollock, N., Letts, L., Bosch, J. and Westmorland, M. (1998) *Guidelines for Critical Review Form: Quantitative Studies*. Ontario: McMaster University [https://alterbiblio.com/content/uploads/2021/09/mcmasters_quantitative-review.pdf].

Leufstadius, C., Nilsson, L. and Hovbrandt, P. (2024) Experiences of meaningful occupation among diverse populations: a qualitative meta-ethnography, *Scandinavian Journal of Occupational Therapy*, 31: 2294751 [https://doi.org/10.1080/11038128.2023.2294751].

Leung, W. (2001) How to design a questionnaire, *Student BMJ*, 322: 0106187 [https://doi.org/10.1136/sbmj.0106187].

Levac, D., Colquhoun, H. and O'Brien, K.K. (2010) Scoping studies: advancing the methodology, *Implementation Science*, 5: 69 [https://doi.org/10.1186/1748-5908-5-69].

Lincoln, Y.S. and Guba, E.G. (1985) *Naturalistic Inquiry*. Beverley Hills, CA: Sage.

Lindberg, C., Fagerstrom, C., Sivberg, B. and Willman, A. (2014) Concept analysis: patient autonomy in a caring context, *Journal of Advanced Nursing*, 70 (10): 2208–2221.

Lizarondo, L., Stern, C., Carrier, J., Godfrey, C., Rieger, K., Salmond, S. et al. (2024) Chapter 8: Mixed methods systematic reviews (2020), in E. Aromataris, C. Lockwood, K. Porritt, B. Pilla and Z. Jordan (eds.) *JBI Manual for Evidence Synthesis*, JBI [https://jbi-global-wiki.refined.site/space/MANUAL/355829175/8.+Mixed+methods+systematic+reviews].

Lyman, B., Jacobs, J., Hammond, C. and Gunn, M. (2019) Organisational learning in hospitals: a realist review, *Journal of Advanced Nursing*, 75 (11): 2352–2377.

McArthur, A., Klugarova, J., Yan, H. and Florescu, S. (2020) Chapter 4: Systematic reviews of text and opinion, in E. Aromataris and Z. Munn (eds.) *JBI Manual for Evidence Synthesis*, JBI.

McCallum, K., Jackson, D., Walthall, H. and Aveyard, H. (2019) Qualitative end of life research with bereaved individuals: looking at current practice. A focused mapping review and synthesis, *Nurse Researcher*, 27 (3): 14–19.

McGowan, J., Sampson, M., Salzwedel, D.M., Cogo, E., Foerster, V. and Lefebvre, C. (2016) PRESS peer review of electronic search strategies: 2015 guideline statement, *Journal of Clinical Epidemiology*, 75: 40–46.

McKibbon, K.A., Wilczynski, N.L. and Haynes, R.B. (2006) Developing optimal search strategies for retrieving qualitative studies in PsycINFO, *Evaluations and the Health Professions*, 29 (4): 440–454.

Majid, U. and Vanstone, M. (2018) Appraising qualitative research for evidence synthesis: a compendium of quality appraisal tools, *Qualitative Health Research*, 28 (13): 2115–2131.

Marmot, M.G., Altman, D.G., Cameron, D.A., Dewar, J.A., Thompson, S.G. and Wilcox, M. (2012) The benefits and harms of breast cancer screening: an independent review, *The Lancet*, 380 (9855): 1778–1786.

Mattioli, S., Farioli, A., Cooke, R.M.T., Baldasseroni, A., Ruotsalainen, J., Placidi, D. et al. (2012) Hidden effectiveness? Results of hand-searching Italian language journals for occupational health interventions, *Occupational and Environmental Medicine*, 69 (7): 522–524.

Mays, N., Pope, C. and Popay, J. (2005) *Details of approaches to synthesis – a methodological appendix to the paper: Systematically reviewing qualitative and quantitative evidence to inform management and policy making in the health field.* Technical Report. Ottawa and London: Canadian Health Services Research Foundation and NHS Service Delivery and Organisation R&D Programme [https://researchonline.lshtm.ac.uk/id/eprint/19432/].

Methley, A.M., Campbell, S., Chew-Graham, C., McNally, R. and Cheraghi-Sohi, S. (2014) PICO, PICOS and SPIDER: a comparison study of specificity and sensitivity in three search tools for qualitative systematic reviews, *MNC Health Services Research*, 14: 579 [https://doi.org/10.1186/s12913-014-0579-0].

Mills, K., Waite, M., McGeach, L. and Aveyard, H. (2024) *A focussed mapping review of patient participation, shared decision making and informed consent.* Paper presented to the RCN International Research Conference, Newcastle.

Mimmo, L., Woolfenden, S., Travaglia, J. and Harrison, R. (2019) Partnerships for safe care: a meta-narrative of the experience for the parent of a child with intellectual disability in hospital, *Health Expectations*, 22 (6): 1199–1212.

Minary, L., Trompette, J., Kivits, J., Cambon, L., Tarquinio, C. and Alla, F. (2019) Which design to evaluate complex interventions? Toward a methodological framework through a systematic review, *BMC Medical Research Methodology*, 19: 92 [https://doi.org/10.1186/s12874-019-0736-6].

Mitchell, S., Bennett, K., Morris, A., Slowther, A.-M., Coad, J. and Dale, J. (2020) Achieving beneficial outcomes for children with life-limiting and life-threatening conditions receiving palliative care and their families: a realist review, *Palliative Medicine*, 34 (3): 387–402.

Mounce, G., Greenway, K., Brueton, V. and Aveyard, H. (2024) Approaches to concept analysis: issues for consideration, *Journal of Advanced Nursing*, 81 (5): 2243–2245.

Mulrow, C.D. (1994) Systemic reviews: rationale for systematic reviews, *British Medical Journal*, 309 (6954): 597–599.

Munn, Z., Peters, M.D.J., Stern, C., McArthur, A. and Aromataris, E. (2018) Systematic review or scoping review? Guidance for authors when choosing between a systematic or scoping review approach, *BMC Medical Research Methodology*, 18: 143 [https://doi.org/10.1186/s12874-018-0611-x].

Niela-Vilén, H., Axelin, A., Salantera, S. and Melender, H.L. (2014) Internet-based peer support for parents: a systematic integrative review, *International Journal of Nursing Studies*, 51 (11): 1524–1537.

Niskala, J., Kanste, O., Tomietto, M., Miettunen, J., Tuomikoski, A.-M., Kyngäs, H. et al. (2020) Interventions to improve nurses' job satisfaction: a systematic review and meta-analysis, *Journal of Advanced Nursing*, 76 (7): 1498–1508.

Noblit, G.W. and Hare, R.D. (1988) *Meta-Ethnography: Synthesizing Qualitative Studies* (Qualitative Research Methods, vol. 11). London: Sage.

Noyes, J. (2010) Never mind the quality, feel the depth! The evolving role of qualitative research in Cochrane intervention reviews, *Journal of Research in Nursing*, 15 (6): 525–534.

Noyes, J. and Popay, J. (2007) Directly observed therapy and tuberculosis: how can a systematic review of qualitative research contribute to improving services? A qualitative meta-synthesis, *Journal of Advanced Nursing*, 57 (3): 227–243.

O'Mathuna, D. P. (2010) Critical appraisal of systematic reviews, *International Journal of Nursing Practice*, 16 (4): 414–418.

Page, M.J. and Moher, D. (2016) Mass production of systematic reviews and meta-analysis: an exercise in meta-silliness?, *Millbank Quarterly*, 94 (3): 515–519.

Papaioannou, D., Sutton, A., Carroll, C., Booth, A. and Wong, R. (2010) Literature searching for social science systematic reviews: consideration of a range of search techniques, *Health Information and Libraries Journal*, 27 (2): 114–122.

Pawson, R. and Tilley, N. (1997) An introduction to scientific realist evaluation, in E. Chelimsky and W.R. Shadish (eds.) *Evaluation for the 21st Century: A Handbook*. Thousand Oaks, CA: Sage.

Pawson, R., Greenhalgh, T., Harvey, G. and Walshe, K. (2005) Realist review: a new method of systematic review designed for complex policy interventions, *Journal of Health Services Research and Policy*, 10 (suppl. 1): 21–34.

Peoples, H., Satink, T. and Steultjens, E. (2011) Stroke survivors' experiences of rehabilitation: a systematic review of qualitative studies, *Scandinavian Journal of Occupational Therapy*, 18 (3): 163–171.

Popay, J., Roberts, H., Sowden, A., Petticrew, M., Arai, L., Rodgers, M. et al. (2006) *Guidance on the conduct of narrative synthesis in systematic reviews*. ESRC Methods Programme. Swindon: ESRC [https://www.researchgate.net/publication/233866356_Guidance_on_the_conduct_of_narrative_synthesis_in_systematic_reviews_A_product_from_the_ESRC_Methods_Programme].

Pope, C. and Mays, N. (2006) Synthesising qualitative research, in C. Pope and N. Mays (eds.) *Qualitative Research in Health Care*. Oxford: Blackwell.

Pope, C., Mays, N. and Popay, J. (2007) *Synthesising Qualitative and Quantitative Health Evidence: A Guide to Methods*. Maidenhead: Open University Press.

Preston, N.J. (2004) *The development of a nursing intervention for the management of malignant ascites*, PhD dissertation, Institute of Cancer Research, London.

Prochaska, J.O., Norcross, J.C. and DiClemente, C.C. (1994) *Changing for Good*. New York: William Morrow.

Qian, F., Yao, D., Shi, H., Tung, T.-H. and Bi, D. (2025) Barriers to healthcare professionals screening, recognizing, and managing delirium in the adult patients receiving specialist palliative care: a mixed-methods systematic review, *BMC Palliative Care*, 24: 28 [https://doi.org/10.1186/s12904-024-01634-w].

Richardson, W.S. (1998) Ask, and ye shall retrieve [EBM note], *Evidence-Based Medicine*, 3 (4): 100–101.

Rock, S., Michelson, D., Thomson, S. and Day, C. (2015) Understanding foster placement instability for looked after children: a systematic review and narrative synthesis of quantitative and qualitative evidence, *British Journal of Social Work*, 45 (1): 177–203.

Rodgers, B.L. (1989) Concepts, analysis and the development of nursing knowledge: the evolutionary cycle, *Journal of Advanced Nursing*, 14 (4): 330–335.

Rodgers, B.L. (2000) Concept analysis: an evolutionary view, in B. Rodgers and K. Knafl (eds.) *Concept Development in Nursing: Foundations, Techniques, and Applications*, 2nd edition. Philadelphia, PA: W.B. Saunders.

Rogers, A., Popay, J. and Williams, G. (1996) *Rationale and standards for the systematic review of qualitative literature in health services research.* Paper presented at the Third International Interdisciplinary Qualitative Health Research Conference, Bournemouth.

Ryan, F., Coughlan, M. and Cronin, P. (2007) Step-by-step guide to critiquing research. Part 2: qualitative research, *British Journal of Nursing*, 16 (12): 738–744.

Rycroft-Malone, J., McCormack, B., Hutchinson, A.M., DeCorby, K., Bucknall, T.C., Kent, B. et al. (2012) Realist synthesis: illustrating the method for implementation research, *Implementation Science*, 7: 33 [https://doi.org/10.1186/1748-5908-7-33].

Saba, M., Diep, J., Saini, B. and Dhippayom, T. (2014) Meta-analysis of the effectiveness of smoking cessation interventions in community pharmacy, *Journal of Clinical Pharmacy and Therapeutics*, 39 (3): 240–247.

Sackett, D.L., Rosenberg, W.M.C., Gray, J.A., Haynes, R.B. and Richardson, W.S. (1996) Evidence based medicine: what it is and what it isn't, *British Medical Journal*, 312 (7023): 71–72.

Sand-Jecklin, K. and Sherman, J. (2013) Incorporating bedside report into nursing handoff, *Journal of Nursing Care Quality*, 28 (2): 186–194.

Sandelowski, M., Docherty, S. and Emden, C. (1997) Focus on qualitative methods. Qualitative metasynthesis: issues and techniques, *Research in Nursing and Health*, 20 (4): 365–371.

Schulz, K.F. and Grimes, D.A. (2002) Allocation concealment in randomised trials: defending against deciphering, *The Lancet*, 359 (9306): 614–618.

Schulz, K.F., Chalmers, I., Hayes, R.J. and Altman, D.G. (1995) Empirical evidence of bias: dimensions of methodological quality associated with estimates of treatment effects in controlled trials, *Journal of the American Medical Association*, 273 (5): 408–412.

Seers, K. (2007) Evaluating complex interventions, *Worldviews on Evidence-Based Nursing*, 4 (2): 67–68.

Shin, K.R., Kim, M.Y. and Chung, S.E. (2009) Methods and strategies utilized in published qualitative research, *Qualitative Health Research*, 19 (6): 850–858.

Sibbald, B. and Roland, M. (1998) Understanding controlled trials: why are randomised controlled trials important?, *British Medical Journal*, 316 (7126): 201.

Skelton, J. and Edwards, S.L.J. (2000) The function of the discussion section in academic medical writing, *British Medical Journal*, 320 (7244): 1269–1270.

Smiddy, M.P., O'Connell, R. and Creedon, S.A. (2015) Systematic qualitative literature review of health care workers' compliance with hand hygiene guidelines, *American Journal of Infection Control*, 43 (3): 269–274.

Smith, J. and Noble, H. (2025) Understanding sources of bias in research, *Evidence-Based Nursing*, March, 28 (3): 137–139.

Smith, M.L. and Shurtz, S. (2012) Search and ye shall find: practical literature review techniques for health educators, *Health Promotion Practice*, 13 (5): 666–669.

Sollaci, L.B. and Pereira, M.G. (2004) The introduction, method, results and discussion (IMRAD) structure: a fifty-year survey, *Journal of the Medical Libraries Association*, 92 (3): 364–367.

Spencer, L., Ritchie, J., Lewis, J. and Dillon, L. (2003) *Quality in qualitative evaluation: a framework for assessing research evidence*. National Centre for Social Research, Occasional papers series 2. London: Government Chief Social Researcher's Office and Cabinet Office [https://www.gov.uk/government/publications/government-social-research-framework-for-assessing-research-evidence].

Stern, P. and Harris, C. (1985) Women's health and the self-care paradox: a model to guide self-care readiness – clash between the client and nurse, *Health Care for Women International*, 6 (1/3): 151–163.

Sun, W., Innes, K., Yu, S. and Collie, A. (2025) Persistent changes of nurses' practices and working conditions in high acuity settings in the post-pandemic era: a qualitative meta-aggregation, *Journal of Advanced Nursing* [https://doi.org/10.1111/jan.16887].

Sutton, A., Clowes, M., Preston, L. and Booth, A. (2019) Meet the review family: exploring review types and associated information retrieval requirements, *Health Information and Libraries Journal*, 36 (3): 202–222.

Taylor, G., McNeill, A., Girling, A., Farley, A., Lindson-Hawley, N. and Aveyard, P. (2014) Changes in mental health after smoking cessation: systematic review and meta-analysis, *British Medical Journal*, 348: g1151.

Thiselton, A.C. (2012) Reception theory, H.R. Jauss and the formative power of scripture, *Scottish Journal of Theology*, 65 (3): 289–308.

Thomas, J. and Harden, A. (2008) Methods for the thematic synthesis of qualitative research in systematic reviews, *BMC Medical Research Methodology*, 8: 45 [https://doi.org/10.1186/1471-2288-8-45].

Thomas, J., Sutcliffe, K., Harden, A., Oakley, A., Oliver, S., Rees, R. et al. (2003) *Children and healthy eating: a systematic review of the barriers and facilitators*, EPPI Report, Social Science Research Unit, Institute of Education, University of London [https://eppi.ioe.ac.uk/cms/Portals/0/PDF%20reviews%20and%20summaries/Summary.pdf?ver=2006-03-03-164136-833].

Thorne, S. (2017) Meta-synthetic madness: what kind of monster have we created, *Qualitative Health Research*, 27 (1): 3–12.

Thorne, S., Jensen, L., Kearney, M.H., Noblit, G. and Sandelowski, M. (2004) Qualitative metasynthesis: reflections on methodological orientation and ideological agenda, *Qualitative Health Research*, 14 (10): 1342–1365.

Thouless, R.H. and Thouless, C.R. (1953) *Straight and Crooked Thinking*. Sevenoaks: Hodder & Stoughton.

Tong, A., Sainsbury, P. and Craig, J. (2007) Consolidated criteria for reporting qualitative research (COREQ): a 32-item checklist for interviews and focus groups, *International Journal for Quality in Health Care*, 19 (6): 349–357.

Tong, A., Flemming, K., McInnes, E., Oliver, S. and Craig, J. (2012) Enhancing transparency in reporting the synthesis of qualitative research: ENTREQ, *BMC Medical Research Methodology*, 12: 181 [https://doi.org/10.1186/1471-2288-12-181].

Toye, F., Seers, K. and Barker, K. (2014) A meta-ethnography of patients' experiences of chronic pelvic pain: struggling to construct chronic pelvic pain as 'real', *Journal of Advanced Nursing*, 70 (12): 2713–2727.

van Hoorn, R., Kievit, W., Booth, A., Mozygemba, K., Lysdahl, K.B., Refolo, P. et al. (2016) The development of PubMed search strategies for patient preference for treatment outcomes, *BMC Medical Research Methodology*, 16: 88 [https://doi.org/10.1186/s12874-016-0192-5].

Wallace, M. and Wray, A. (2021) *Critical Reading and Writing for Postgraduates*, 4th edition. London: Sage.

Walsh, D. and Downe, S. (2005) Meta-synthesis method for qualitative research: a literature review, *Journal of Advanced Nursing*, 50 (2): 204–211.

Walsh, D. and Downe, S. (2006) Appraising the quality of qualitative research, *Midwifery*, 22 (2): 108–119.

Walsh, S.A., Walker, S.B. and Wirihana, L.A. (2024) Preregistration nursing students' motivation for speaking up for patient safety: an integrated literature review, *Nurse Education Today*, 140: 106291 [https://doi.org/10.1016/j.nedt.2024.106291].

Webster, N.L., Oyebode, J.R., Jenkins, C., Bicknell, S. and Smythe, A. (2020) Using technology to support the emotional and social well-being of nurses: a scoping review, *Journal of Advanced Nursing*, 76 (1): 109–120.

West, R. (2006) *Theory of Addiction*. Oxford: Blackwell.

Whiting, P., Wolff, R., Mallett, S., Simera, I. and Savovic, J. (2017) A proposed framework for developing quality assessment tools, *Systematic Reviews*, 6: 204 [https://doi.org/10.1186/s13643-017-0604-6].

Whittemore, R. and Knafl, K. (2005) The integrative review: updated methodology, *Journal of Advanced Nursing*, 52 (5): 546–553.

Whittemore, R., Chase, S. and Mandle, C. (2001) Validity in qualitative research, *Qualitative Health Research*, 11 (4): 522–537.

Wilczynski, N.L., Marks, S. and Haynes, R.B. (2007) Search strategies for identifying qualitative studies in CINAHL, *Qualitative Health Research*, 17 (5): 705–710.

Wiles, R., Crow, G. and Pain, H. (2011) Innovation in qualitative research methods: a narrative review, *Qualitative Research*, 11 (5): 587–604.

Wong, G., Greenhalgh, T., Westhorp, G., Buckingham, J. and Pawson, R. (2013a) RAMESES publication standards: realist syntheses, *BMC Medicine*, 11: 21 [https://doi.org/10.1186/1741-7015-11-21].

Wong, G., Greenhalgh, T., Westhorp, G., Buckingham, J. and Pawson, R. (2013b) RAMESES publication standards: meta-narrative reviews, *BMC Medicine*, 11: 20 [https://doi.org/10.1186/1741-7015-11-20].

Wong, S.S., Wilczynski, N.L. and Haynes, R.B., for the Hedges Team (2004) Developing optimal search strategies for detecting clinically relevant qualitative studies in MEDLINE, *Medinfo*, 11 (1): 311–316.

Zitomer, M.R. and Goodwin, D. (2014) Gauging the quality of qualitative research in adapted physical activity, *Adapted Physical Activity*, 31 (3): 193–218.

Index

Page numbers with 't' are tables; in italics are figures.

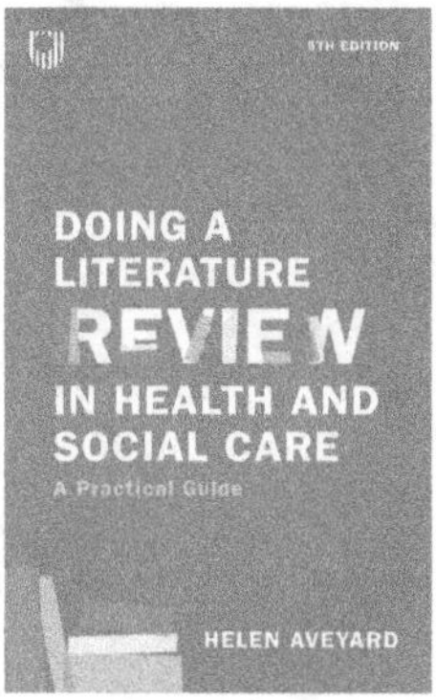

Doing a Literature Review in Health and Social Care: A Practical Guide

Helen Aveyard

Fifth Edition

ISBN: **9780335251940** (Paperback)

eISBN: 9780335251957

2023

This best-selling book, now in its fifth edition, is a step-by-step guide to doing a literature review for students in all areas of health and social care. It is essential reading for all those doing their undergraduate dissertation or any study that involves doing a literature review.

The new edition maintains its signature 'can do' approach and provides a practical guide to doing a literature review from start to finish. This book includes:

- **A broad and updated range of real life examples of how to overcome challenges in the process**
- **Tips on how to get your question right**
- **Updated guidance on following a clear search strategy for relevant literature using the appropriate technology**
- **Brand new and accessible chapter summaries**
- **An expanded guide for the application of critical appraisal tools**
- **An increased emphasis on presenting your findings or using them in practice**

Doing a Literature Review in Health and Social Care is vital reading for anyone new to reviewing and presenting evidence in a review

www.mheducation.co.uk

OPEN UNIVERSITY PRESS

McGraw Hill

www.ingramcontent.com/pod-product-compliance
Lightning Source LLC
LaVergne TN
LVHW022212200926
848481LV00006B/1933